Which Diet is Best for Me?

A Quick & Easy Guide for Women Over 50 to Lose Weight, Eat Better & Feel Healthier

Robin Bartko, M.S.

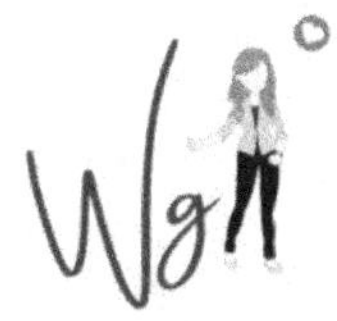

WellnessGirlfriend.com

Dedication

For all my 50 and older girlfriends and girlfriends I can't wait to meet who want to get their gusto back and make positive changes to live their best lives...

Contents

Acknowledgements

I want to thank my husband, Dennis, for helping me put this book together by answering all my computer questions (not my forte), formatting, running ideas by, and supporting me during the time of writing this book. This book would not have come to completion without him. Also, a great big thank you to my dear friend, Lisa Morrow, for her editing skills and my niece, Hillary McCarthy, for creating the awesome book cover. Lastly, I want to thank all my girlfriends and family who gave me feedback on topics to write about, reviewed book cover ideas, and encouraged me. You all rock!

Disclaimer

The information in this book has not been evaluated by the Food and Drug Administration. It is for education purposes only. It is not intended to treat, cure, or prevent disease or illness. Readers should not ignore or delay in getting medical or mental health advice from their personal physician or mental health provider.

CHAPTER ONE

Introduction

You are probably reading this book because you want to lose a few pounds or more, you are confused by all the weight loss information out there (let's face it, the info in the media and social media can be confusing), you are interested and intrigued in learning more about various diets or you have struggled with weight loss before. For many of you, the dreaded dropping a few pounds has truly been a roller coaster that you want to get off of. By reading this book, you are in the right place. I will guide and support you in finding the best healthy weight loss plan for you. A weight loss plan that helps you feel better about yourself and have those jeans not feel so snug. However, most of all, I am here to help you feel better and be healthier as you age. If you have any questions while taking this journey, please feel free to email me at Robin@WellnessGirlfriend.com. Girlfriend, I am here for you!

Weight loss is more than just the number that we dread seeing on the scale, it truly is about getting a healthier you! As we age, who wants to be limited by what we can do because our health is poor, we don't feel up to doing things, or we have a bunch of unexpected medical bills to pay? Many women, over the age of 50, really believe that they cannot lose weight anymore due to their genetics, metabolism, stress levels, etc. In my experience, in health coaching and health education, I have found that this is not true for the majority of women. It may be just one or two things they are doing not so well that are sabotaging their weight loss. For me, years ago, I was stress eating a lot in the evening after my kids went to bed. I had a child with challenges and my anesthesia of choice to tame my emotions was eating at night (lots of diet sodas and snack mix). Once I got my stress and healthier choices of foods down, weight loss took place. I must confess, I still like a good snack in the evening, but it is now a healthier and low-calorie option that still t astes delicious.

I am here for you along this journey of finding the best diet plan for you that works. A diet plan that makes you feel more alive, have more energy, and not dread getting on that scale on Monday morning after the weekend.

As I mentioned, at any time you have a question, feel free to email me at Robin@Well nessGirlfriend.com. Sometimes, I get a lot of emails, so please allow 48 hours for me to respond. If you need more guidance, we can set up a virtual time to chat.

CHAPTER TWO

Getting Started

Making the Commitment

Many women truly feel unsettled and bad about their weight. They talk about it a lot, hate to look in the mirror at times, hate how their clothes fit, and so on...yet still don't make any progress on reducing their weight and improving their wellness. They often feel defeated before they even start. Having a deep heart-to-heart conversation with yourself on why you want to lose weight is imperative. A good way to start is to share your plans with friends and supportive family. Have people hold you accountable if you don't comply during your weight loss journey. A helpful technique is recording your feelings by journaling as well. Also, hold <u>yourself</u> accountable. So, it was a friend's birthday and you were trying to be polite and you ate a piece of vanilla bean cake with chocolate icing. It was only a small piece. You didn't want to be rude by not having any. Don't beat yourself up over it! However, the next day, get out there for a long walk or get on the treadmill to make up for it. Admit you got off track and get back on that horse right away and do better. Self-observation is a good thing, but reminding yourself and taking action to not follow the same patterns is even better.

Connecting with your "Why"

Connecting with your **"why"** is an important place to start with. Why do you want to lose weight and live a life you are proud of? A life where you feel more comfortable in your own skin. You know what I mean, a life where you are not embarrassed to wear that adorable dress or special blouse to a wedding or your son's college graduation.

Here are some examples:

- I want to look good at my reunion

- I want to not be embarrassed in a swimsuit

- I want my ex to take a double take the next time they see me

- I have a wedding or graduation coming up and I want to feel relaxed, confident, and good!

<u>Why do you want to lose weight?</u>

Now, take time and write down three reasons why you want to lose weight ...

1.

2.

3.

Put this list on your refrigerator door and/or bathroom mirror and remind yourself each day. Say them out loud!

Here is some more information to get started....

Carbs, Proteins, and Fats

Carbs:

Most people know what carbs are. Carbs can be that awesome piece of homemade bread, a sweet donut, a big bowl of granola, cereal, or even a sweet potato. We all know some skinny girl who eats three donuts at work or church and doesn't gain a pound. The reality is that some women process carbs differently than others. However, for the majority of us, lots of carbs can result in us taking a double take in the mirror of our stomach, thighs, and rump. Carbs are sugar, fiber, and starches. Regardless of the type of carb, they eventually break down as sugar. Healthy carbs include non-starchy vegetables and low-glycemic fruits (think berries) which have awesome minerals, nutrients, and fiber. Carbs have 4 calories per gram.

Proteins:

Protein is very important especially as we age. Protein helps us feel fuller, build muscle mass, and regulate our immune system. These are all important things as we age, especially since we tend to lose muscle tone every year. This was especially true since Covid hit when activity levels have been less. Protein is made from amino acids which our body cannot make by itself so we must consume them. Protein has 4 calories per gram.

Fats:

Fats are needed for our brain, hair, skin, and nail health which are all very important as we age. Omega 3 fats (think salmon and other cold-water fish, walnuts, flaxseeds, etc.) in particular are needed as they are anti-inflammatory, which is helpful with autoimmune disorders and joint pain. Fat is needed to help absorb vitamins as A, D, E, and K. If you try to go on a basic no-fat diet, you are not doing yourself any favors. Fats have 9 calories per gram.

A little more to get you started...

What's the not-so-skinny deal with the Standard American Diet?

For women, the Standard American Diet aka SAD tends to be a very high-carb, high-fat, low-protein diet. A high-carb diet in particular can cause insulin spikes and blood sugar problems among other health risks. If your doctor tells you that you are prediabetic or diabetic, you must take that knowledge and make changes to your diet and lifestyle so that you can have a better quality of life as you age. Don't you want to travel, play with your grandkids or nieces and nephews, and, do your favorite hobbies instead of going to the doctors all the time and using your hard-earned money on medical bills and prescriptions?

One last thing to get you started...

Pick a diet that has foods you like

This may sound kind of silly or weird, but it really is important to pick a diet with foods you like. For example, if you know that you just cannot give up cheese, then a diet such as the Paleo diet is not for you. You can just skip that one and look at the other diet options. You know your preferences and tastes the best, so it is important to consider that.

CHAPTER THREE

My Wellness Journey

I wanted to share my wellness journey and how I lost over 96 pounds and have kept it off. My road to wellness started when my husband and I adopted our youngest son from overseas. Even though my new son was a chubby, bald toddler with gorgeous blue eyes when we adopted him, he came home with some health challenges. One of his biggest challenges was the intestinal giardia he came home with which is often caused by the poor water supply in his home country. To put it politely, it was a crappy mess. My son had loose bowels and I couldn't even run into Target with him without having to run to the bathroom to change yet another diaper. I had read about giardia before we adopted him and knew there was a risk that he may have it and he did. Also, I had read previously that there was a nasty-tasting medicine to give him that would clear it up quickly. After being diagnosed with giardia, my son's pediatrician put him on the nasty-tasting medicine and said it should be cleared up in a few weeks. Unfortunately, my son's gut was a mess and a few weeks turned into 9 months. Not only did I have to give him the medication for quite a while, but I also had to learn a lot about which foods he could tolerate, which foods help restore his gut, and which foods he was willing to eat. It was not easy getting a toddler that I was trying to bond with to comply with this process. I learned a lot about how food affected his body. Fortunately, my son is now grown, and you would never guess how his now 6-foot-5-inch body went through that and he can now eat all kinds of food. Like many young adult men, he loves Chipotle.

Fast forward, after that journey with my son, I decided to learn more about nutrition and stress management. I earned a certificate in health coaching and studied in detail over 100 different diets. At that same time, I decided to make an effort to improve my health by losing weight and working on my stress management. After trial and error, I found a diet that worked for me, and I lost over 96 pounds. Also, I will share in this book, some of my health issues with migraines and severe digestive issues too. For over 30 years I was overweight and struggled with losing weight. Also, the interesting thing is that I have had digestive issues later in life, which created challenges at times in keeping weight on. Go figure, it is a weird feeling that I have been on both sides of the coin on this issue. To continue to keep up with my wellness and control my weight, I learned to make my version of the diet personalized so that it works for me as a lifestyle way of eating.

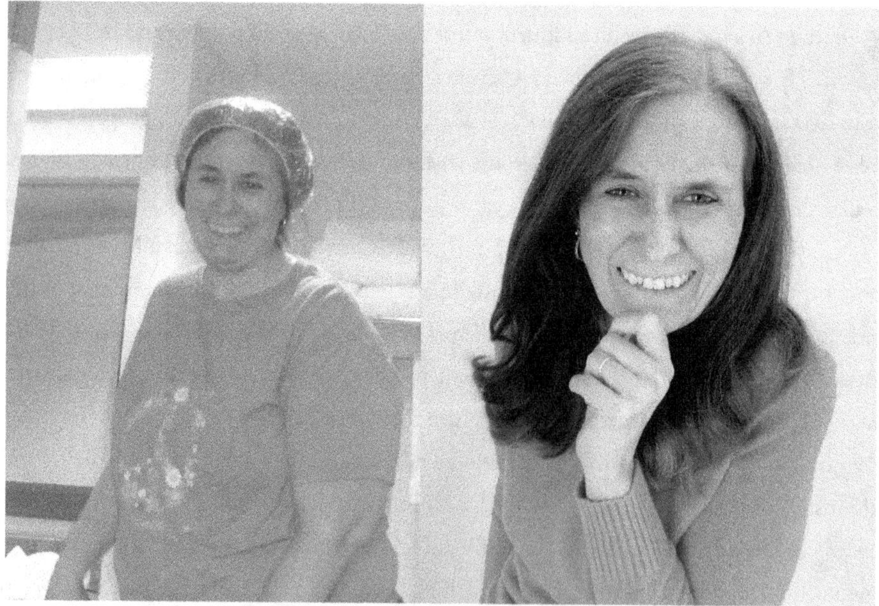

Me, before (left) and after (right) my weight loss

Later, when my three kids got older, I followed my passion and earned my master's degree in health promotion where I do health education, coaching, and promotion. I have presented and participated in a variety of programs from taking *Girl Scout* troops on healthy grocery store tours to giving seminars on breast cancer prevention to women, suicide prevention, reducing screen addiction, nutrition, etc. to name a few. That is how I became known as the *Wellness Girlfriend.*

As I side note, I do believe in having some cheat meals or snacks. Life would be very sad not to ever enjoy your favorite piece of cheesecake or eat your favorite chips again. I don't believe in that. The key is to make it a special occasion and not a daily occurrence. Good food is meant to be enjoyed! and as your Wellness Girlfriend, I am not recommending taking that away from you.

Wishing my best to you to improve your wellness. Now let's get started on learning about the various diets...

CHAPTER FOUR

Anti-inflammatory Diet

My favorite anti-inflammatory diet is by Dr. Andrew Weil. Dr. Weil is a well-respected, Santa-bearded, Harvard-trained doctor. Dr. Weil is known in the wellness circuit for being good-natured and knowledgeable, as well as having an infectious smile of contentment (he has that Santa-type personality quality too!). He is a big believer in stress management. (Let's face it gals, we can eat all the broccoli in the world, but if our stress isn't in check, our life can be miserable, and the pounds can jump on fast). Dr. Weil has lived in places such as India and Greece and is the founder of the *Andrew Weil Center for Integrative Medic*ine in Arizona. He has an anti-inflammatory diet that is very popular and nutrient-dense. By nutrient-dense, I mean that the foods in his plan have a lot of sound, good nutrition in them and are very good quality. He bridges the gap between integrative and conventional medical wisdom. He, also, has a popular skincare line and a restaurant chain called *True Food Kitchen*.[1] He has a lot of great diet and lifestyle information online that may be of interest to you. This is a diet I tend to use when I coach someone with inflammation challenges or an autoimmune disease such as Multiple Sclerosis, Lupus, or Rheumatoid Arthritis.

To share a little more about inflammation. Some inflammation is not a bad thing, but excessive inflammation can present itself with symptoms such as muscle and joint pains and aches, digestive issues, skin rashes, etc.[2] If your doctor tells you that your CRP is high, then what they are referring to is your C-reactive protein (CRP). If your CRP is high, then you typically have high levels of inflammation.[3] High sugar, processed food, and refined carbs are usually associated with inflammation. In other words, if you are a gal who loves three bowls of high-sugar cereal (not that any of us have ever done that) in the morning or for dinner, then you may have inflammation. Moderation is key. As I mentioned before, I am not a believer in giving up your favorite foods, but I am a believer in good nutrition the majority of the time. Getting back to inflammation, it is associated with diseases such as Alzheimer's, Asthma, Cancer, Heart disease, Type 2 Diabetes, PCOS, and Autoimmune disorders such as Rheumatoid Arthritis, MS, and Lupus.[4] Both Livestrong and Dr. Weil's websites have great anti-inflammatory meal ideas to check out. The resource links are at the end of the chapter. I must confess, that some of the recipes are really yummy!

Who is this diet best for?

Someone who has an autoimmune disease, autoimmune tendencies, or autoimmune diseases that run in their family.

For example, my mom had severe rheumatoid arthritis. She had the crippling kind where her hands were cradled in, and she had multiple knee replacements. As an adult, I often think about how difficult it was for her to deal with her illness and raise a house full of kids. As a kid, I didn't think about that. Isn't hindsight something to ponder as we age? Anyway, although the genetics for me, of having her illness is fairly low, I want to increase my odds of not having her destiny as I age so I follow a diet similar to this.

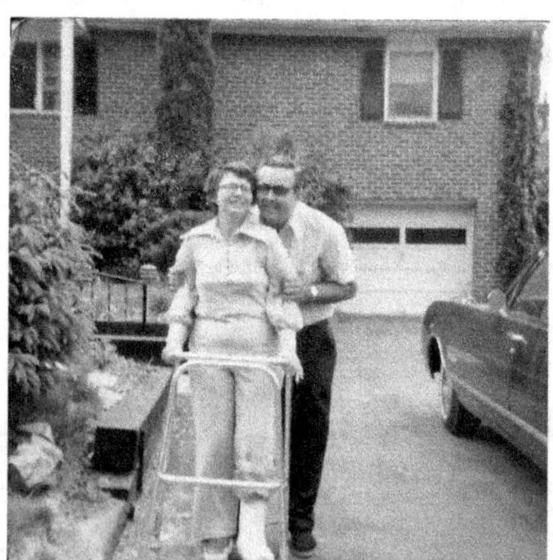

My Mom and Dad

Here is a list of who this diet is best for

- Someone who likes a lot of vegetables and fruit

- Someone who likes seafood

- Someone who is focusing on their bone/joint health

- Someone who enjoys a glass of red wine or two

- Someone with likes tea

- Someone who does not want to give up pasta

- Someone who likes to grocery shop, meal prep, plan, and cook

- Someone who likes to focus on the quality of food

- Someone who has a budget for supplements

Who is this diet <u>not</u> best for?

- Someone who wants rapid weight loss

- Someone who is short on time and can't do meal prep

- Someone who has digestive issues with fructose. This diet tends to have about 3 to 4 servings of fruit per day (although modifications can be made for this)

- Someone who prefers not to spend money on supplements and organic food

- Someone who eats out a lot as cooking is required

- Someone who does not do well eating a fair amount of fat

- Someone who has issues with digesting beans and legumes

- Someone who has issues with dairy

What foods are typically eaten on the Anti-Inflammatory Diet?[5]

- Vegetables-especially organic as well as cooked mushrooms

- Fruits such as berries, apples, pears, and grapes (not tropical fruits as they tend to be higher glucose)

- Eggs

- Lean meats such as skinless chicken and grass-fed beef

- Nuts and Seeds

- Healthy fats such as olive oil, avocados, and walnuts

- Fish and seafood as sockeye salmon, sardines, and black cod

- Dairy as natural cheeses and yogurt (low sugar ones)

- Whole soy as edamame, tofu, and soy nuts

- Whole grains such as brown, wild, and basmati rice as well as quinoa and steel-cut oats

- Pasta cooked al dente

- Beans and lentils

- Spices and herbs especially turmeric, ginger, cinnamon, and chili peppers

What can you drink?

- Teas as white, green, and oolong (unsweetened)

- Water with lemon or a splash of fruit juice

- Red Wine

What treats can you eat?

- Dark chocolate

- Fruit sorbet

- Unsweetened dry fruit

- Red Wine

What foods can't you eat?[6]

- No added sugar foods-this includes packaged foods such as cereal, donuts, white loaf bread, etc. (sorry gals, *Little Debbie's* snack cakes are a no-go)

- Some oils as palm oil and hydrogenated oils

- Artificial sweeteners such as aspartame are discouraged

- Soda

- Sports drinks

Robin's take on this diet

This diet has a lot of great qualities. It focuses on vegetables and fruits, which provide a lot of good nutrition. I have found that this diet is very helpful for those with muscle stiffness and joint pain. It does require meal prep, diligent grocery shopping, planning, and cooking. I think the quality of the food tends to be better on this diet compared to many other diets. This diet may be more difficult to get started with but as a long-term food lifestyle, it is great. It can be expensive with organic food and supplements, but so are bags of chips and boxes of cereal! Frozen food can help reduce costs too!

Resources:

- **Dr. Weil's Food Pyramid:**

  - https://www.drweil.com/wp-content/uploads/2017/06/dr-weils-anti-infla mmatory-diet-and-food-pyramid-print.pdf

- **Dr. Weil's newsletter**:

  - https://www.drweil.com/newsletter/

- **US News diet review:**

  - https://health.usnews.com/best-diet/anti-inflammatory-diet/review

- **Dr. Weil YouTube:**

  - *"The TOP FOODS To Eat To Reduce Inflammation & LOSE BELLY FAT"* with Andrew Weil, MD — A video on healthy aging — https://www.you tube.com/watch?v=MHTO8wDbrKs

  - *"Integrative Health for Optimal Aging"* with Andrew Weil, MD — https ://www.youtube.com/watch?v=zPZocdqp8JI

- **Recipes:**

  - https://www.drweil.com/diet-nutrition/recipes/

  - https://www.livestrong.com/article/13721269-anti-inflammatory-recipes/

---

1. Healthy Lifestyle Brands, LLC. (2019, August). *About Andrew Weil, M.D.* DrW eil.com. https://www.drweil.com/health-wellness/balanced-living/meet-dr-weil/a bout-andrew-weil-m-d/

2. Cleveland Clinic. (2021, July 28). *Inflammation: What is it, causes, symptoms & treatment.* Cleveland Clinic. https://my.clevelandclinic.org/health/symptoms/21 660-inflammation

3. Wikimedia Foundation. (2023, August 9). *C-reactive protein.* Wikipedia. https://e n.wikipedia.org/wiki/C-reactive_protein

4. U.S. Department of Health and Human Services. (2021, April 28). *Inflammation.* National Institute of Environmental Health Sciences.

5. Weil, A. (2017). dr-weils-anti-inflammatory-diet-and-food-pyramid-print.pdf. Weil Lifestyle LLC. https://www.drweil.com/wp-content/uploads/2017/06/dr-weils -anti-inflammatory-diet-and-food-pyramid-print.pdf

6. Leaf Group. (n.d.). *Dr. Weil's anti-inflammatory diet: What to eat and avoid.* LI VESTRONG.COM. https://www.livestrong.com/article/13721067-dr-weil-anti -inflammatory-diet/

CHAPTER FIVE

Counting Calories Diet

The counting calories diet is very much like it sounds. The premise is you must count calories for weight loss. There is some controversy over this as some foods digest slower than others, our genetics are unique, and our metabolisms vary. However, I must say that I think and know that counting calories is crucial in weight loss. I often hear women say they count calories, and they don't lose weight. From my experience, if you indeed count calories accurately, and eat and drink fewer calories than your body requires then most women will lose weight regardless of their age.

Who is this diet best for?

- Someone who needs to lose 15 pounds or less

- Someone who likes math and doesn't mind counting calories or using an app like *Lose It*

- Someone who has a goal in mind. For example: I want to lose 10 pounds by my daughter's or niece's wedding.

- Someone who tends to comply and stay on task for a set period of time

Who is this diet <u>not</u> best for?

- Someone who tends to be impulsive and often eats what they see

- Someone who hates tracking calories

- Someone who eats junk food the majority of the time

- Someone who eats most of their food by takeout or restaurants. This is because the calories and portion sizes may be underestimated on the menu, especially with condiments added

- Someone who is taking medications that may deter weight loss (consult your doctor on this one)

What foods can you eat on this diet?

You can eat any foods on this diet, but to lose weight and have good nutrition, I would recommend eating a lot of non-starchy vegetables, lean protein, and keeping the carbs to a minimum. Non-starchy vegetables in particular tend to be low in calories.

How to get started

Determine how many calories your body needs daily. This is your starting point. I like using the *Mayo Clinic Calorie Calculator*,[1] which can be accessed using the below link:

The Calorie Calculator will ask you your height, current weight, age, gender, and activity level. You enter it and then it gives you how many calories you need to maintain your current weight. So for example, if you are a 5-foot 4-inch 55-year-old woman who weighs about 165 pounds and is a little active, you need about 1,850 calories to maintain your weight.

https://www.mayoclinic.org/healthy-lifestyle/weight-loss/in-depth/calorie-calculator/it t-20402304

There are 3,500 calories in a pound. Therefore, if you want to lose 1 pound per week, you need to reduce your calories by 500 calories a day. In the above example, you would take 1,850 less 500=1,350 calories per day.[2] Of course, you can burn some additional calories by exercise activity as well.

Counting Calories Example

Calories required per day *(use calorie calculator)*   1,850

Calories eaten per day   - 1,350

____

Calories not used   500

500 calories per day X 7 days = 3,500 calories = 1 pound

It is very important to remember that muscle burns more calories than fat and as we age, we tend to lose muscle. The skinny is that you can lose almost 100 more calories per pound of muscle in a 24-hour day [compared to fat tissue].[3] Therefore, we should focus on exercise that tends to focus on resistance training to increase the muscles in our bodies. Resistance training includes activities such as modified push-ups, stability balls, hip lifts as well as things like raking leaves.[4] If you have limitations as knee issues then ask your local gym like the *YMCA* for guidance on which exercises are best for you. Have them model the exercise for you and then try it. Keep a log of your activity and stay consistent in doing it. List the activities on your phone or paper and make a check mark each time you do it.

Write it out on paper or use your app to create meal plan ideas. I find it best to have 3 sample meal ideas each for breakfast, lunch, and dinner.

Make your grocery list:

Keep your list on your phone or a piece of paper in your pocket for easy reference.

Shop for your groceries. Remember that non-starchy vegetables tend to be low in calories so you can eat a lot of them. Don't worry if you are not a big veggie lover, just pick out 3 or 4 that you like. If you hate kale but love green beans or cucs then search the internet for great recipes for the vegetables that you like. Don't make eating vegetables a brutal task for yourself.

Start eating and use your app or a piece of paper to log your caloric intake -include everything that touches your lips.

The biggest issues I see with people who count calories and don't lose weight are the following:

- **They underestimate their calorie consumption** – That extra squirt of ketchup or salad dressing can really add up. That mini bite-size chocolate bar that wasn't recorded in the calorie count matters too! Those small bags of chips count too! The 100-calorie packs of snacks matter too when you eat 2 or 3 of them a day. That 2nd glass of wine was small, but it matters too! Remember if it touches the lips it can add to the hips. Count all foods and drinks consumed.

- **They drink their calories in soda, juices, and smoothies** – I often hear women say that they really don't eat that much but don't understand why they can't lose weight. Believe it or not, when I review what they are eating, it is often true. However, an important thing to look at is how much soda, juices, and smoothies that are being consumed. A can of soda can have 8 to 12 teaspoons or more of sugar in it. Orange soda tends to be more. Apple and other juices in bottles are very high in sugar and calories too! Smoothies can be made lower in calories, but servings of fruit for flavor need to be limited to low glycemic fruits like berries and ½ cup size. Check out the following chart.

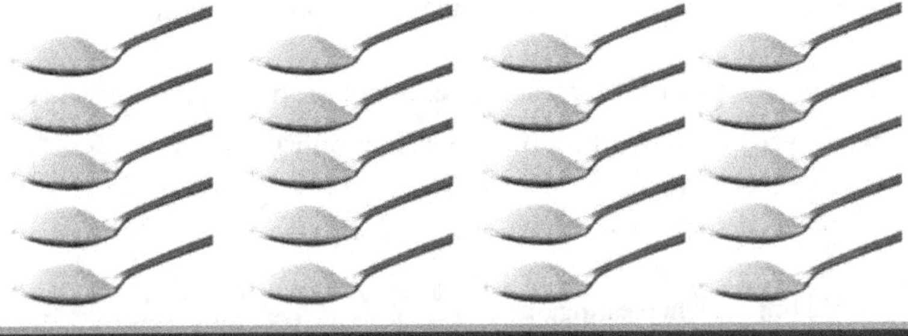

- **They guestimate their calories and often underestimate** them – This is something that I am guilty of. What the heck, I'm a health coach and should know this stuff. I know that a medium-sized banana has around 100 calories, an egg has around 70 calories, and 3 ounces of chicken is around 200 calories, but I still tend to underestimate calories in other foods. It is especially easy to do this if you are eating out. That delicious salad at your favorite restaurant had almonds and avocado on it, or your grilled chicken sandwich had lettuce tomato, and lots of mayo on it. The best way I have found to truly count your calories is to use an app like *Lose It, My Fitness Pal, Chronometer, or Fitbit.* These apps are really good and fairly low-cost. To start, don't worry so much about the carbs, protein, or fats, just track your calories.

- **They blame their poor metabolism** – I think we all have had friends who eat way more than us and still stay skinny. Some women indeed have a better metabolism than others but, in my experience, the majority of women can lose weight if they count their calories. If this is a concern of yours, a great way to increase your metabolism is to build muscle in your body.

If you have now decided to start watching your calories, here are some tips I have learned along the way to get you rolling...

Tips for reducing calories

- Try using small size plates or bowls for each meal

- Drink one or two glasses of water an hour before your meal

- Keep the chips and other snack foods out of the house or locked in a cabinet where you cannot see them (men aren't the only visual ones)

- If you get dessert, share it with a friend

- Avoid buffets when eating out

- Get salad dressing on the side (non-creamy ones tend to have less calories)

- Take time to eat slowly and don't multitask (it's easy to be on your phone, watch TV, and shove that food in oh so fast). Take time to savor and enjoy your food. Notice what you like and don't like about the meal. Don't eat foods you don't enjoy!

- When eating out, be specific about your requests. For example, can they make the food with little or no butter? can they put a sauce on the side? can they put ½ the meal in a take-home back before you start to eat? In the past, I used to feel bad asking the server to do this, but now it is part of my routine and works out well.

- Review the menu of a restaurant before you go so you can look at the lower-calorie options. Most restaurants have calories on the menu or online to check out.

- Eat lots of veggies and some protein. Avoid the bread bowl or crackers. You may want to request not to even bring the bread bowl to the table.

Robin's take on this diet

I have found that counting calories is very important and that most women can lose weight by counting calories. It can be effective short term, however, it may not be as nutritious as other dietary practices because you can eat whatever you want. If your daughter or granddaughter is getting married in a month and you want to drop some weight before then it may be a quick diet for you. However, long term it is important to have a good nutritional diet that includes vegetables, fruits, healthy protein, and whole grains.

Resources:

- **Calorie Calculators and more:**

    ○ Calorie calculator - Mayo Clinic — https://www.mayoclinic.org/healthy-lifestyle/weight-loss/in-depth/calorie-calculator/itt-20402304

    ○ Body Weight Planner - NIDDK (nih.gov) — https://www.niddk.nih.gov/bwp

    ○ Seafood Watch -To learn more about quality seafood choices or if you have a concern about mercury in fish — https://www.seafoodwatch.org/recommendations/search?query=%3Abuy%3BGre

- **Speeding Metabolism over 40:**

    ○ "Speeding Up Metabolism After 40: Live Q&A" with Dr. Neal Barnard — https://www.youtube.com/watch?v=BdusT4vUFKM

    ○ How Much Sugar Is in Coke and Other Sodas? – verywellfit.com — https://www.verywellfit.com/guess-how-much-sugar-is-in-a-can-of-soda-2506919#citation-9

- **Apps:**

- Lose It! — https://www.loseit.com/

  - MyFitnessPal — https://www.myfitnesspal.com/

  - Chronometer — https://cronometer.com/

- **Recipes:**

  - Healthy Recipes – Joy Bauer (joybauer.com) — https://joy-bauer.com/healthy-recipe/recipes-index/
    I like this site because if you have leftover items in your house like bananas that you want to use up, you can search by type of food or type of meal. For example, if you are tired of the same old breakfast, you can search for breakfast ideas.

  - Recipes Search – Dr. Axe (draxe.com) — https://draxe.com/recipes-search/#results
    I like this one because you can search by diet preference, kind of meal, and ingredients.

---

1. Mayo Foundation for Medical Education and Research. (n.d.). *Calorie calculator.* Mayo Clinic. https://www.mayoclinic.org/healthy-lifestyle/weight-loss/in-depth/calorie-calculator/itt-20402304

2. American Academy of Family Physicians. (2003, January 1). *What it takes to lose weight.* American Family Physician.

3. You + Health. (n.d.). *1lb of Fat vs. 1lb of muscle: Let's clear up the misconceptions for maximal weight-loss.* You + Health. https://youplushealthusa.com/blog/1lb-of-fat-vs-1lb-of-muscle-lets-clear-up-the-misconceptions-for-maximal-weight-loss3/

CHAPTER SIX

Vegan Diet

I often hear women say they aspire to eat a vegan or vegetarian diet. They think it is great, and admire women who do it (dang that Christy Brinkley still looks good!), but have not tried it. I, also, have known women who think they eat a healthy vegan or vegetarian diet, but they actually eat a lot of junk food, lots of cheese, unhealthy carbs, but no meat. A healthy vegan diet includes grains, beans, pasta, nuts, seeds, vegetables, and fruits. A true vegan diet does <u>not</u> include meat, fish, any animal by-products, honey, dairy, or eggs. A Vegetarian diet is very similar to a vegan diet but does include dairy, honey, and eggs.

One of the leading experts on Vegan Diets is Dr. Neal Barnard (pronounced Barn-ard). I remember his name by saying he does not eat a Barn Yard without the "y." He is a Clinical researcher and Professor at George Washington University. His fields of expertise include doing research and writing books on how diet affects weight, hormones, Type 2 Diabetes, etc.[1] He has even conducted a study on the dreaded hot flashes.[2] His diet recommendations include low-fat and plant-based options. He is a strong believer in prevention, which I am a big fan of as well. Also, he is the President of a nonprofit called *the Physician Committee for Responsible Medicine.* This nonprofit is well respected, does an extensive amount of research, and has done some very interesting and impactful studies.[3] I was blessed to have met Dr. Barnard at a presentation at my local library.

After treatment for breast cancer, one of my best friends changed to a vegetarian diet and has followed it for over 20 years. My heart still sinks sometimes remembering when she got diagnosed at age 39 and had 4 young kids. Have you ever noticed how life can be so unfair at times? Anyway, back to the diet.

Who is this diet best for?

- Someone who needs to lose weight and wants to eat vegetables

- Someone who loves vegetables and fruits

- Someone who has strong convictions on protecting the treatment of animals, antibiotic use in animals, and the environment

- Someone who likes to cook and prepare food

- Someone who will review menu items online before eating out

- Someone who wants to not only lose weight but eat a healthier nutrient-dense diet as well

- Some women who want to lose weight as they are at risk for breast cancer or breast cancer reoccurrence. Not sure you know this, but losing weight is one of the top 5 recommendations for breast cancer prevention.[4] Last year I did a presentation on this at my local church. Cutting down on booze helps too!

Who is this diet <u>not</u> best for?

- Someone who doesn't want to eliminate junk food

- Someone who frequents a lot of burger restaurants or steak houses

- Someone who hates vegetables

- Someone who needs to eat Gluten Free Diet, as many Vegan products like veggie burgers often have gluten

- Someone whose doctor recommends a very low-carb diet

- For someone with a digestive disease like IBS or candida as too much fiber or juicing can cause discomfort.[5] Consult with your doctor on that one.

- Someone with a soy or nut allergy

- Someone with low B12

What foods are typically eaten on a Vegan diet?

- Vegetables-all

- Fruits -all

- Nuts and Seeds

- Plant-based oils such as vegetable, olive, avocado, or walnut

- Whole soy as edamame, tofu and soy nuts

- Whole grains such as brown, wild, and basmati rice as well as quinoa and steel-cut oats

- Most Pastas

- Beans and Lentils

- Spices and Herbs

- Plant-based milks such as almond, coconut, or oat milk

- Plant-based yogurts like almond or coconut

- Nutritional yeast (which has a cheesy flavor). It is often tasty on popcorn

What can you drink?

- Water and most flavored waters

- Most coffees, but if you add cream it will not be unless a nondairy creamer is used

- Most teas, but check the labels

- Some alcohol – this is a tricky one as many alcoholic drinks have ingredients in them such as gelatin, whey, dairy, etc. which are not vegan.[6] Label reading is a must.

What treats?

- Most Dark chocolates-check the labels. Milk chocolate tends not to be vegan

- Fruit sorbet

- Unsweetened dry fruit

- Some alcohols -check the labels[7]

What foods can't you eat?

- Dairy as milk, butter, margarine, cheese, and ice cream

- Honey

- Eggs

- Meat which includes beef, pork, lamb, chicken, turkey, and duck

- Seafood

- Whey products

- Products with gelatin

- Most mayonnaise products

Robin's take on this diet

In my experience, I have found that success with a vegan diet depends on how it is done and based on each individual. I have known women who changed to a vegan diet due to their health provider's recommendations. They truly eat a large amount of vegetables, fruits, and whole grains and are say they feel healthier. I, also, have known women who follow a vegan diet but eat a lot of unhealthy foods such as chips, high-sugar items, and lots of carbs. The critics of vegan diets often are concerned about the lack of B12 (which you can supplement with) and the amount of carbs that are eaten as high-carb diets are often not recommended for women with conditions such as type 2 diabetes. Many studies have shown that meat consumption is tied to higher cancer risk, especially red meat.[8] I have found that men, in particular, are not fond of a vegan diet because they really don't want to give up meats such as steaks, ribs, and sausages. My husband is definitely one of those men. Suggesting a vegan diet to him is like asking him if he likes to get a tooth pulled!

Important!

Most vegans need to supplement with B12.[9] B12 is essential for nerve and blood function in our bodies.

If you are a gal who wants to try a vegan diet, I would recommend working with a dietician, or health coach or using an online program to create balanced meals and snacks and to make sure you get enough healthy protein, carbs, and fat. There are a lot of great recipes on the internet for the vegan diet. See the recipe resources at the end of this chapter.

Even if you don't want to become a complete vegan, you can consider eating more vegetables, fruits, less processed foods, and whole grains for some of your meals. Some women try to limit meat only for dinner or only eat it a few times a week. One thing to keep in mind is that you may want to focus on eating more non-starchy vegetables than fruit as they tend to be lower in calories, which aids in weight loss.

Resources:

- **Bio on Dr. Barnard**

    ◦ https://www.pcrm.org/about-us/staff/neal-barnard-md-facc

- **Dr. Barnard's nonprofit**

    ◦ https://www.pcrm.org/

- **Dr. Barnard's nonprofit article on Hot Flashes** is very interesting

    ◦ https://www.pcrm.org/clinical-research/fighting-hot-flashes-with-diet

- **B12**

    ◦ https://www.vegansociety.com/resources/nutrition-and-health/nutrients/vitamin-b12/what-every-vegan-should-know-about-vitamin-b12

- **Recipes**

    ◦ https://www.pcrm.org/good-nutrition/plant-based-diets/recipes

- **21-day quick starter challenge**

    ◦ https://www.pcrm.org/vegankickstart

- **Podcast on cancer-fighting foods**

    ◦ https://www.pcrm.org/news/exam-room-podcast/cancer-fighting-foods

1. Wikimedia Foundation. (2023, July 15). *Neal D. Barnard*. Wikipedia. https://en.wikipedia.org/wiki/Neal_D._Barnard

2. Physicians Committee for Responsible Medicine. (n.d.). *Fighting hot flashes with Diet*. Physicians Committee for Responsible Medicine. https://www.pcrm.org/clinical-research/fighting-hot-flashes-with-diet

3. Wikimedia Foundation. (2023, July 15). *Neal D. Barnard*. Wikipedia. https://en.wikipedia.org/wiki/Neal_D._Barnard

4. American Cancer Society. (2022, September 19). *Lifestyle-related breast cancer risk factors*. American Cancer Society. https://www.cancer.org/cancer/types/breast-cancer/risk-and-prevention/lifestyle-related-breast-cancer-risk-factors.html

5. Silver, N. (2021, April 20). *Vegan diet for IBS: Research, effectiveness, and tips*. Healthline. https://www.healthline.com/health/ibs/vegan-diet-for-ibs Medically reviewed by Kim Chin, RD, Nutrition.

6. Meixner, M. (2020, January 30). *Is alcohol vegan? A complete guide to beer, wine, and Spirits*. Healthline. https://www.healthline.com/nutrition/is-alcohol-vegan Katherine Marengo served as medical reviewer vs. editor.

7. Meixner, M. (2020, January 30). *Is alcohol vegan? A complete guide to beer, wine, and Spirits*. Healthline. https://www.healthline.com/nutrition/is-alcohol-vegan Medically reviewed by Katherine Marengo, LDN, R.D., Nutrition

8. Genkinger, J. M., & Koushik, A. (2007, December 11). *Meat consumption and cancer risk*. PubMed Central. https://www.ncbi.nlm.nih.gov/pmc/articles/PMC2121650/

9. Niklewicz, A., Smith, A. D., Smith, A., Holzer, A., Klein, A., McCaddon, A., Molloy, A. M., Wolffenbuttel, B. H. R., Nexo, E., McNulty, H., Refsum, H., Gueant, J.-L., Dib, M.-J., Ward, M., Murphy, M., Green, R., Ahmadi, K. R., Hannibal, L., Warren, M. J., … CluB-12. (2023, April). *The importance of vitamin B12 for individuals choosing plant-based diets*. European journal of nutrition. https://www.ncbi.nlm.nih.gov/pmc/articles/PMC10030528/

CHAPTER SEVEN

Keto Diet

You've probably have heard of the Keto Diet or a variation of it. Perhaps you have known some girlfriends or family members who have lost weight with it and have said they are not even hungry. There are many variations of the Keto Diet, which can include healthy and unhealthy options. It is important to eat healthier for your long-term well-being and to lose weight. There is the diary-free Keto Diet, MCT Keto Diet, Calorie Restricted Keto Diet, Cyclical Keto Diet, etc. to name a few. For this discussion, I'm going to introduce you to the Standard Keto Diet aka SKD.

The skinny on what is the Keto Diet

Basically, the Keto Diet is a very high-fat, low-carb diet. Daily, it typically is about 70% fat, 25% protein, and 5 % carbs.[1] Eating higher-fat meals can put your body in ketosis. Ketosis is where your body burns fat instead of glucose. Ketosis can also be achieved by intermittent fasting such as eating all your calories within an 8-hour time frame daily.[2] The carb intake is usually about 20-50 **net carbs** per day. Net carbs are the carbs less the fiber.[3] For example, ½ cup of raspberries has approximately 7 carbs and 4 grams of fiber (they are fiber all-stars) so the net carbs are only 3 net carbs. This is why raspberries are a preferred fruit on the Keto diet. Many people do find success in losing weight on the Keto Diet. The Keto diet was originally developed to combat medical conditions such as epilepsy and research concluded that it can reduce seizures.[4] The Keto diet has been used especially with children and adults who do not respond to typical medications. You may have heard from friends who have kids with autism with seizures and they are trying a Keto diet for their child.

The Standard American Diet tends to be very high in carbs which often does not help with weight loss and managing conditions as Type 2 Diabetes. However, keep in mind that counting calories still matters for weight loss. If you eat a large quantity of high-fat meals, you will most likely gain weight.

So, What Foods Can I eat on a Keto Diet?

Here is a list of whole food options:

- Meats: Bacon, Beef, Chicken, Lamb, Pork, Turkey especially dark meat

- Seafood and Fish

- Nuts/Seeds

- High-fat dairy such as butter, cream, cheese, unsweetened yogurt, and cottage cheese

- Eggs

- Oils: Olive, Avocado, Coconut

- Berries such as Strawberries and Raspberries

- Avocados

- Non-starchy vegetables such as zucchini, broccoli, bell peppers, leafy greens such as spinach, kale, and collard greens

- Unsweetened plant milks such as soy, almond, or coconut

What foods to avoid

- High carb foods

- Rice

- Bread

- Starchy vegetables like potatoes and sweet potatoes, corn, winter squashes such as acorn or butternut

- Beets

- Onions (moderation only)

Who is this diet best for?

- Someone who likes to food prep and try new recipes

- Someone who has time to learn the diet

- Someone who wants to feel full and satisfied after eating (aka satiety)

- Someone who wants to potentially lose weight at a slightly faster pace than other diets

- Someone who likes to review the menu online prior to eating out

Who is this diet <u>not</u> best for?

- Someone who has chronic digestive challenges, especially with eating fat.[5] I am one of those people that has struggled with that. Too much fat (even the healthy ones like avocadoes) sometimes results in a stomachache and headache

- Someone with pancreatic and gallbladder issues[6]

- Someone who wants to lose a fair amount of weight in just a week or two. This diet takes time to learn, implement, and adjust for your body. However, it could take 3-8 weeks to see real results.

- Someone who is not willing to give up most carbs. This includes whole grains, cereals, pasta, granola, and even some starchy vegetables. Typically the Keto diet has a limit of 20-50 carbs daily. That is around 10 to 15 carbs per meal. After reading the labels, you will be able to determine that it is a very small amount of carbs and some women find that they cannot comply with that few carbs long-term.

- Someone who just can't give up the bread basket, as most breads have lots of carbs

- Someone who hates meat (although Keto can be done without meat it is much more difficult to sustain)

- Someone who has been diagnosed by a doctor or is consulting with a doctor that they have hypoglycemia[7] (low blood sugar).

- Someone who is pregnant or breastfeeding and is new to Keto (I know we are beyond that age but good to know for our daughters and nieces)

- Someone who is looking for a quick diet to learn and implement. The Keto Diet takes time to be successful

- Someone who doesn't like to cook much or meal prep.

- Someone who cannot give up alcohol.[8] Most Booze has a lot of carbs and can raise blood sugar levels

Some challenges people may have with the Keto Diet[9]

- Muscle cramps from electrolyte imbalances. However, often times this can be balanced out with careful dietary practices.

- Thirst

- Feelings of being drained or low energy

- Headaches

- Kidney Stones

Robin's take on this diet

The Keto Diet can be successful for a lot of people. I am not a big fan of it for long-term use unless one's doctor recommends it. I have found that many women have a hard time eating a lot of meat and giving up so many carbs. Women just aren't used to eating so much high-fat food and really miss their carbs. This makes it hard to sustain. I think it depends on how much weight someone needs to lose, compliance, and planning. Also, an important thing to consider is if you have any health conditions that may make following the Keto Diet difficult.

Resources:

- **App:**

  ○ Carb Manager — https://www.carbmanager.com/

- **Book:**

  ○ *Keto QuickStart* by Diane Sanfilippo — https://a.co/d/bIAfL7p
  If you want to start a Keto Diet, this is a great place to start. It is excellent! It has full-color pictures of recipes, keto meal ideas, and Keto Swops. Keto Swops are really great so that you can learn what keto foods to have instead of the old favorites you have become accustomed to. For example, if you are a cereal lover, you can swap it for a flavored chia oatmeal. If you love crackers, you can have cheese crisps instead. Also, there is a helpful Keto Food List that shows the net carbs, protein, and fat of each food item. I love the Lemon Caper Salmon recipe in this book I think you will find this book is worth

every penny! You can find it on Amazon using the above link.

---

1. Harvard T.H. Chan School of Public Health. (n.d.). *Diet Review: Ketogenic Diet for weight loss*. The Nutrition Source. https://www.hsph.harvard.edu/nutritionsourc e/healthy-weight/diet-reviews/ketogenic-diet/

2. Fletcher, J. (2023, January 5). *How to get into ketosis faster*. Medical News Today. https://www.medicalnewstoday.com/articles/324599#7-strategies

3. Spritzler, F. (2023, May 15). *How to calculate net carbs*. Healthline. https://www. healthline.com/nutrition/net-carbs

4. Cleveland Clinic. (2020, October 6). *Ketogenic diet (keto diet) for epilep- sy*. https://my.clevelandclinic.org/health/treatments/7156-ketogenic-diet-keto-di et-for-epilepsy

5. Mouw, M. (2019, May 22). *Low fat vs. high fat– which diet is better for the gut microbiota?*. Gut Microbiota for Health. https://www.gutmicrobiotaforhealth.co m/low-fat-vs-high-fat-which-diet-is-better-for-the-gut-microbiota/

6. Helms, N. (2023, January 3). *Ketogenic diet: what are the risks?*. At the Fore- front. https://www.uchicagomedicine.org/forefront/health-and-wellness-articles /ketogenic-diet-what-are-the-risks

7. Spoke, C., & Malaeb, S. (2020, April 18). *A case of hypoglycemia associated with the ketogenic diet and alcohol use*. Journal of the Endocrine Society. https://www.ncbi .nlm.nih.gov/pmc/articles/PMC7278276/

8. Icahn School of Medicine at Mount Sinai. (n.d.). *Diabetes and alcohol*. Mount Sinai Health System. https://www.mountsinai.org/health-library/selfcare-instructions/ diabetes-and-alcohol

9. Masood, W., Annamaraju, P., Khan Suheb, & M. Z., Uppaluri, K. R. (2023, June 1 6). *Ketogenic diet*. In: StatPearls [Internet]. https://www.ncbi.nlm.nih.gov/book s/NBK499830/

CHAPTER EIGHT

Low Carb Diet

You may be considering a low-carb diet right now because you have prediabetes, type 2 diabetes, or know someone who you are concerned about who has diabetes. It is not uncommon for doctors to advise their patients to follow a low-carb diet to lose weight or for health reasons. The challenge is that many women really don't know how to get started with this so I will fill you in on it.

A low-carb diet typically is a low-carb, low-fat, lean protein, and low-sugar diet. Depending on your weight loss goals, genetics, metabolism, and health concerns, you and your medical provider can determine how many carbs <u>per day</u> to aim for. I have found that most women who fill ½ their plate with non-starchy vegetables, a small amount of carbs, and small portions (like the size of a playing card) of lean proteins do have success in losing weight on this diet. You do not have to give up all carbs, but do need to be more mindful of the number of carbs you eat and the portion sizes. For example, fewer donuts and more portion-controlled whole grains or one bowl of cereal instead of two.

How to get started on a Low Carb Diet?

Get the tempting foods out of your house and away from your desk or workplace

You may have heard that it is best not to take a recovering alcoholic to a bar, the same applies here. Don't have high-carb cookies, cakes, crackers, breads, donuts, cereals, or chips in your house. Get them out of your eyesight so you are not tempted. If you have other family members who are not on board, put the high-carb foods in a cabinet that is locked so that you don't have access to them.

Instead, fill your refrigerator with lots of non-starchy vegetables such as baby carrots, peppers, and cucumber slices. I like to keep mine in glass mason jars, so they are easy to see when I open the refrigerator. Keep proportioned packs (think small sandwich bags) of snacks such as whole grain crackers available.

Have low-sugar, tasty drinks available

Sodas are a big issue with the Standard American Diet. It is one thing to have a sugary soda once in a while when you go out to eat. It is another thing to drink two or more sodas per day. Sodas have no nutritional benefits, are high in calories, and don't help with your long-term energy levels. There is a lot of controversy about the use of artificial sweeteners in diet sodas.[1] You may have heard about Splenda in the news recently. Research has shown that soda consumption is linked to obesity.[2] I often hear women say they don't eat that much and often it is true, but they do drink a lot of sodas, smoothies, juices, expressos, lattes, and ice coffees (I know Dunkin Rocks). I must confess I still love to go occasionally to *Dunkin* and *Starbucks*, but I now know how to order something that is still tasty and has less sugar and carbs. For example, at Starbucks, you can order an herbal tea with stevia or an almond milk hot chocolate with only one or two pumps of syrup. I really like the passion tea with stevia. Make sure you are specific when ordering.

Consider having water with a splash of juice, sparkling water, or flavored purchased water. Save that big Latte for after your diet. You don't have to give it up forever, just until you achieve your weight loss goal.

Read labels or get an app

Reading labels or getting an app to track your carbs is important. Most women are shocked when they see that the little 100-calorie pack of crackers or cookies has 30 plus carbs. They really did not know how high in carbs many items are. Also, be sure to look at ingredients on package labels. If the package has an ingredient that ends in "ose", it tends to have sugar in it. Words like sucrose, fructose, maltose, etc.

What carbs and other foods can I eat?

Complex carbs are the best to eat. This includes, in small portions, chickpeas (there are some really great recipes to spice them up), beans, lentils, oats, brown rice, and quinoa. Be sure to check serving sizes on packages or use your app to check the carb count.

- Vegetables such as asparagus, green beans, broccoli, cauliflower, carrots, egg-plant, spinach, tomatoes, and zucchini (typically have about 5 carbs per cup raw and ½ cup cooked)

- Whole fruits such as apples, oranges, pears, peaches, bananas (1/2), and berries have about 15 carbs per serving

- Nuts and seeds

- Meat

- Seafood and Fish

Nebraska Medicine has a great chart you can print that shows carb amounts with serving sizes. See the resources section below for more info.[3]

What foods should I avoid or limit?

- Cakes

- Cookies

- Pies

- Bagels

- Chips

- Pretzels

- Bread Baskets

- Booze

Portion size is very important — You can eat chips and pretzels, but who really eats only a few? Also, on desserts, if it is sweet and soft like cakes and cookies, it typically is high carbs.

So how many carbs should I eat daily?

This is a very common question. It really depends on multiple factors as your current weight, height, age, gender, genetics, activity level, etc. Some women choose a very low-carb diet with about 50 carbs per day and others try to stay under 150 carbs per day. A traditional low-carb diet typically has less than 130 grams of carbs per day. The best way is to ask your doctor, nutritionist, health coach, or registered dietitian. That way if you have multiple health concerns (for example, osteopenia and diabetes) they can come up with a plan just for you. Also, you are always welcome to email me at Robin@WellnessGirlfriend.com for some resources.

Another carb issue to remember is that it is often helpful to spread your carbs throughout the day and not all in one sitting. For example, half of an English muffin for breakfast or one slice of bread for lunch instead of a triple high sandwich or burger all at once. Another way to think about it is to instead of eating three bowls of cereal (not that any of us have done that), have just one serving of cereal with some low glycemic fruit like berries and some protein for breakfast. Spreading your carbs out throughout the day is something to get used to but it can be done.

Who is this diet best for?

- Someone whose doctor recommends they follow a low-carb diet which often includes women with type 2 diabetes, prediabetes, nonalcoholic fatty liver disease, heart disease, etc.[4]

- Someone who has time to use an app or count and record their daily carbs

- Someone who likes to check out the menu online items before eating out

- Someone who doesn't want to restrict their carbs as much as on other diets like the Keto diet

Who is this diet <u>not</u> best for?

- Someone pregnant, exercises a lot, or is a performance athlete. Most of us reading this book are not in any of these categories

- Someone who is not willing to give up most carbs. This includes whole grains, Olive Garden breadsticks (they are to die for), cereals, pasta, granola, and even some starchy vegetables.

- Someone who just won't give up the breadbasket, as most breads have lots of carbs.

Robin's take on this diet

A lot of women have success losing weight on this diet short term. If they need to lose 10 pounds or less then they can do it. Also, I see a lot of women who fail at this because they really don't like to count their carbs or don't do it consistently. If you want to try this plan, you must track your calories and carbs to have success. It will get easier once you learn how many carbs are in a food item.

Also, I have found that women who check their blood sugar daily have more success. You can get blood sugar meters fairly cheap on Amazon. After seeing their glucose levels rise, women remember they shouldn't have eaten that huge bowl of popcorn the night before or multiple bags of those 100-calorie cookies or chips.

I would recommend not overthinking this diet. The skinny is to eat a bountiful amount of non-starchy vegetables, a little fruit, some lean protein, a little bit of low-fat dairy, and a small amount of carbs. Most vegetables have carbs, but also fiber which reduces the net carbs. No need to worry too much about counting the carbs in the non-starchy vegetables as you will feel full and can eat a lot of them.

Resources:

- **Nebraska Medicine carb chart**

    - https://www.nebraskamed.com/sites/default/files/documents/Diabetes/2_9212%20Carb%20Counting%20Food%20List.pdf

- **The American Diabetes Association (ADA) website** – has a lot of good information on it. They have an "ask the expert" series of live webinars you can sign up for. Also, they have recorded webinars to watch.

    - https://diabetes.org/

- **The Mayo Clinic Diabetes Diet** is a good program that you can check out. Great books and other resources to help you learn this diet.

    - https://www.mayoclinic.org/diseases-conditions/diabetes/in-depth/diabetes-diet/art-20044295

1. Rios-Leyvraz, M., & Montez, J. (2022). (rep.). *Health effects of the use of non-sugar sweeteners: A systematic review and meta-analysis*. World Health Organization. https://www.who.int/publications/i/item/9789240046429

2. Basu, S., McKee, M., Galea, G., & Stuckler, D. (2013, November). *Relationship of soft drink consumption to global overweight, obesity, and diabetes: A cross-national analysis of 75 countries*. American journal of public health. https://www.ncbi.nlm.nih.gov/pmc/articles/PMC3828681/

3. The Diabetes Center. (n.d.). *Carb Counting Food List*. Nebraska Medicine. https://www.nebraskamed.com/sites/default/files/documents/Diabetes/2_9212%20Carb%20Counting%20Food%20List.pdf

CHAPTER NINE

The MIND Diet

This diet was created by the late Martha Clare Morris with colleagues at Rush University Medical Center. Martha went to Harvard to get her doctorate in epidemiology all while raising her three young children (Wow, you go girl!). She was the director of the *Institute for Healthy Aging at Rush University*. Her goal was to create a nutritional plan that helped with cognitive decline delay. Her son indicated her wishes were not to copywrite or trademark this diet so that it could be used by researchers, scientists, and the public. In addition, she wrote the book, *"Diet for the Mind"*, which includes lots of great recipes that she and her chef daughter created.[1]

Even though you may or may not have heard of this diet before, it has been well-researched. This diet is known as the "good brain" diet so if you are worried about memory loss for yourself or a loved one then this is a diet to check out. I think of it as a blend of the Mediterranean and DASH diets. It is highly plant-based but also includes limited meats and fish/seafood. It is, also, a low-sugar diet where you avoid sweets.

The acronym, **MIND,** stands for "Mediterranean-DASH Intervention for Neurodegenerative Delay."[2]

According to an NIH study, "These data suggest that even modest adherence to the MIND diet score may have substantial benefits for the prevention of AD. By contrast, only the highest concordance to the DASH and MedDiet diets were associated with AD prevention."[3] AD refers to Alzheimer's Disease.

According to Perdue University, "Research shows that the MIND diet can improve brain health and lower your odds of developing conditions like Alzheimer's disease, dementia, and other forms of age-related cognitive decline. In fact, studies have shown that eating certain foods and avoiding unhealthy ones can slow brain aging by 7.5 years."[4]

Gals, if you are worried about memory loss then this is a great diet to check out!

(you know those moments like when you can't find your keys again or you wonder to yourself what you walked into a room for).

What foods do you typically eat on the MIND Diet?

- Vegetables-leafy greens

- Fruits – berries

- Nuts

- Beans

- Fish/Seafood

- Poultry

- Whole grains like oatmeal, quinoa, brown rice, whole wheat pasta

- Olive oil

- Wine (in moderation)

What foods to avoid on the MIND Diet?

- Sweets

- Fried foods (sorry gals, no French fries)

- Red meats

- Cheese

- Butter

Who is this diet good for?

- Someone who is concerned about cognitive delay such as memory loss. Research shows that for people over age 65, one in ten people have Alzheimer's. Also, remember that this statistic may not include those who have cognitive delay, but have not been diagnosed with it.[5] If you want to learn more about Alzheimer's, there is good info to check out in the resource section.

- Someone who is concerned about bone/joint health, diabetes prevention, and heart disease. According to the US News and World Report, this diet was ranked 4 th for these health conditions.[6]

- For someone who wants to follow a Kosher, Halal, or Gluten Free Diet — this diet can accommodate those requirements

- Someone who wants to eat a lot of plant foods

- Someone who doesn't want to give up wine (in moderation)

- Someone who still wants to have an occasional sweet

- Someone who wants to improve their long-term weight loss

- Someone who doesn't want to count carbs or calories as this diet is more per serving based

- Someone who wants a budget-friendly option, as this diet has less meat than many other diets. We all know how pricey meat can be.

Who is this diet <u>not</u> good for?

- Someone who wants rapid or quick weight loss

- Someone who doesn't want to give up red meat and processed meat such as sausage

- Someone who doesn't want to reduce their cheese intake

Robin's take on this diet:

I really like this diet, especially for those who are concerned about memory loss. Often people worry about the physical problems their bodies have as they age. Concerns like bad knees, poor vision, poor hearing, etc. However, cognitive issues are really important to be concerned about too! Why not make it a priority as we age to take care of both our bodies and our minds?

Resources:

- ***2023 Alzheimer's Disease Facts and Figures: Special Report – The Patient Journey in the Era of New Treatments*, Alzheimer's Association**

  - https://www.alz.org/media/Documents/alzheimers-facts-and-figures.pdf

- **Martha Clare Morris' books**

  - https://www.amazon.com/Official-MIND-Diet-Scientifically-Cognitive/dp/031644118X/

  - https://www.amazon.com/Diet-MIND-Science-Alzheimers-Cognitive/dp/0316441155/

- **Meal Plan Ideas and Grocery List**

  - https://thegeriatricdietitian.com/wp-content/uploads/2022/11/MIND

---

1. Megan, G. (2020, March 5). *Martha Clare Morris, Rush researcher who studied link between diet and dementia, dies at 64.* Chicago Tribune. https://www.chicagotribune.com/news/obituaries/ct-martha-morris-obitu ary-20200305-hdklslkgt5gqrnnsrzxvjvj6ye-story.html

2. Sreenivas, S. (2021, September 27). *What to know about the MIND diet.* WebMD. https://www.webmd.com/alzheimers/what-to-know-about-mind-diet

3. Morris, M. C., Tangney, C. C., Wang, Y., Sacks, F. M., Bennett, D. A., & Aggarwal, N. T. (2015, February 11). *MIND diet associated with reduced incidence of Alzheimer's disease.* Alzheimer's & Dementia, Volume 11, Issue 9, p. 1007-1014. https://alz-journals.onlinelibrary.wiley.com/doi/10.1016/j.jalz.2014.11.009

4. Smith, A. (2023, June 15). *Improve your brain and body health: the MIND diet.* Purdue University Extension. https://extension.purdue.edu/news/county/putna m/2023/06/improve-your-brain-and-body-health-the-mind-diet.html

5. Alzheimer's Association. (2023). *2023 Alzheimer's disease facts and figures: special report.* Chicago, IL; Alzheimer's Association. PDF file accessed at: https://www.al z.org/media/documents/alzheimers-facts-and-figures.pdf

6. Esposito, L., & Chien, S. (2023, July 14). *MIND diet.* U.S. News & World Report - Health. https://health.usnews.com/best-diet/mind-diet

CHAPTER TEN

Paleo Diet

The Paleo diet is a diet based on what humans ate in the Paleolithic Era. Some know it as the *Stone Age* Diet. The theory is that it is **not** based on current farming practices. It is a high protein, low carb, unprocessed food diet. Research has shown it is effective in short-term weight loss and may aid with some health issues such as high blood pressure, high cholesterol, high triglycerides, and high glucose issues.[1]

What foods are typically eaten on the Paleo Diet?

- Vegetables – non-starchy

- Fruits-most like apples, berries, cantaloupe, grapes, lemons, oranges, and even watermelon

- Eggs

- Lean meats especially grass-fed

- Nuts and Seeds

- Oils such as Olive and Walnut

- Fish and Seafood as albacore tuna, mackerel, trout, shrimp, salmon

- Spices and Herbs

What can you drink?

- Tea-herbal and matcha

- Coconut Water

- Coffee-black (in moderation)

- Kombucha

- Water

- Wine and other alcohol -in moderation (hey, in ancient times they did it)

What treats?

- Some homemade baked goods that are made from things like arrowroot, al-mond, or coconut flour (Dr. Axe has some great recipes, see the resources section for the link)

- Occasional dark chocolate

What foods can't you eat?

- No grains, legumes lentils, or starchy vegetables — this includes no beans, no peas, no corn, or no potatoes

- No dairy – this includes no milk or cheese

- No added sugar — this includes packaged foods such as cereal, donuts, bread, etc.

- No added salt

- No processed foods

- No soybean, cottonseed (that one is especially bad for you), sunflower, and grapeseed oils

- No artificial sweeteners as aspartame

- No diet sodas or any sodas

- No bacon

- No processed lunch meats

Who is this diet best for?

- Someone who is interested in short-term weight loss.

- Someone who is concerned about improving health issues such as heart disease, high blood pressure, high cholesterol, high triglycerides, or high glucose levels.

- Someone who likes a lot of vegetables and fruit

- Someone who likes fish

- Someone who enjoys an occasional glass of wine

- Someone with likes tea or coffee

- Someone who likes meal prep

- Someone who likes to meal plan and cook

Who is this diet **not** best for?

- Someone who is short on time and can't do meal prep

- Someone who eats a lot of processed foods

- Someone who has digestive issues with processing fat as gallbladder issues.[2]

- Someone who prefers not to spend money on grass-fed meat although the diet can be followed without grass-fed meats.

- Someone who eats out a lot as cooking/meal prep is required

- Someone who refuses to give up dairy as cheese

- Someone who cannot give up grains — note that some people who are not team paleo feel that this diet lacks essential fiber and vitamins

- Someone who wants long-term weight loss

- Someone who is a vegan or vegetarian

Robin's take on this diet

This diet has ranked well for short-term weight loss. However, I have found that many people have difficulty not eating cheese and processed foods. It does require time and energy in meal planning. There are many great and delicious recipe resources available on the internet. Another observation I have noticed is that some people with a lot of migraine headaches and joint aches do better with a lower-carb diet. This is my observation only and not from a big meta-study.

Resources

- **Dr. Axe Paleo Dessert Recipes**

    ◦ https://draxe.com/nutrition/paleo-desserts/

- **Other Paleo Recipes**

    ◦ https://paleogrubs.com/paleo-diet-recipes

- **Paleo Meat Sticks**

  - https://paleovalley.com/store/beef-sticks

- **Book to get started:** *Paleo for Beginners: Essentials to Get Started* by John Chatham

  - https://a.co/d/a6e6ZUp

---

1. Maher, L. (2023, May 25). *The paleo diet and your cholesterol*. WebMD - Cholesterol Management Guide. https://www.webmd.com/cholesterol-management/features/paleo-diet-cholesterol

2. Kubala, J. (2022, May 9). *4 potential side effects of the paleo diet*. Healthline - Nutrition. https://www.healthline.com/nutrition/paleo-diet-side-effects

CHAPTER ELEVEN

DASH Diet

The acronym, DASH, stands for *Dietary Approaches to Stop Hypertension*. This plan is a very well-researched diet that was developed to prevent and reduce hypertension. If you have high blood pressure, you may want to ask your doctor about this diet or your doctor may have already mentioned this diet to you. This diet is a low-fat (especially saturated fat and trans fat), low-sugar, reduced sodium, and high-fiber diet that typically has more protein than the Standard American Diet. The typical diet plate consists of ½ vegetables, ¼ whole grains, and ¼ low-fat protein like beans, lean meat, poultry, turkey or fish.

What foods are typically eaten on the DASH Diet?

- Vegetables

- Fruits

- Whole grains

- Poultry and Turkey (skinless preferred)

- Extra-lean ground beef or sirloins

- Most Fish and Seafood as shrimp, crab, trout, tuna

- Nuts and Seeds

- Beans

- Eggs (limited)

- Low-fat or nonfat dairy

- Oils such as olive, avocado, and canola

What can you drink?

- Tea

- Water

- Coffee

- Diet Soda

- Alcohol in moderation

Sample snacks

- 1/3 cup or less of almonds

- 2 tbs of peanuts (peanuts are actually a legume and I recommend spending the extra few bucks by buying organic on them)

- A few graham crackers

- A small handful of whole grain or wheat crackers

- 1 tablespoon of sunflower seeds

- Fat-free yogurt with no added sugar

What treats?

- There are a lot of treats you can make on the DASH Diet. They often include the following:

- Fruits like strawberries or other berries, peaches or pears, with a small amount of glaze made from a little bit of sugar (I'm talking like a teaspoon or two), maple syrup or honey, or a balsamic vinegar glaze.

- Puddings are often made from yogurt and chia seeds

- Popsicles (oh so good in the summer) and homemade soft serve

There are a lot of great recipes available online, especially on Pinterest and the Mayo Clinic websites. See the recipe resources in the resource section.

What foods to avoid?

- Full-fat dairy

- Fatty meats like hot dogs, bacon, sausage, ham and most beef

- Sugary drinks and soft drinks

- High-sodium packaged food like chips, baked goods, canned soups, premade pizzas, most frozen meals, pretzels, most cereals, and some condiments like k etchup

- Deep-fried foods (sorry gals, French fries, and deep-fried Oreos are out). No worries, I'm not talking forever, just until you reach your health goals and then moderation is the key.

Who is this diet best for?

- Someone who likes to cook and prepare food

- Someone who is consistently willing and interested in reading food labels or using an app

- Someone who is concerned about improving health issues such as heart disease, high blood pressure, high cholesterol, high triglycerides, or high glucose levels[1]

- Someone who likes a lot of vegetables and fruit

- Someone who enjoys an occasional glass of wine

- Someone with likes tea or coffee

- Someone who likes information on a diet that is freely available. NIH has a lot of good info on this diet. See the resource section for more info.

- Vegans and Vegetarians can follow this diet with some substitutions

Who is diet <u>not</u> best for?

- This diet tends to be more a lifestyle diet than a short-term weight loss diet and some people don't want to commit to it long-term

- Someone who has potassium or phosphorus issues. I would consult with your doctor on this one. Also, research shows that those with chronic kidney disease, liver disease, and those on medications such as renin-angiotensin-aldosterone system antagonists should avoid the DASH diet.[2]

- Someone who is short on time and can't do meal prep

- Someone who hates to food track as it is important to track portion sizes and number of portions daily. This diet doesn't necessarily track calories, but portion size is very important.

- Someone who eats a lot of processed foods especially since many processed foods have a lot of sodium. Especially beware of the high sodium in frozen dinner meals.

- Someone who may have fructose digestive issues as many fruits are high in fructose. However, berries tend to be less so.

- Someone who prefers support groups either online or in person with their diet. There are some online groups but fewer than many other diets. However, there are dieticians, nutritionists, and health coaches who can help with this.

Robin's take on this diet

This diet has ranked very well according to the US News and World Report survey on the best diets especially for people with high blood pressure or high cholesterol.[3] There is a fair amount of meal prep and planning so if you are short on time, prefer packaged foods or hate to cook, you may have a big learning curve. There are many great and delicious recipe resources available on the net. If you struggle with high blood pressure, this is a diet to discuss with your doctor.

Resources

- **Recipes**

  - **The Mayo Clinic** – The Mayo Clinic website has a lot of great recipes. The artichoke dip is to die for!

    - https://www.mayoclinic.org/healthy-lifestyle/recipes/dash-diet-recipes/rcs-20077146

  - **The Everyday DASH Diet Cookbook by Marla Heller, MS, RD** – This is a great DASH Diet cookbook.

    - https://a.co/d/6ncaofA

  - **DashDiet.net** – On the dashdiet.net website you can select by meal type like breakfast or dessert.

    - http://thedashdiet.net/

- **More info on the DASH Diet**

  - https://www.nhlbi.nih.gov/files/docs/public/heart/new_dash.pdf

- **App:**

  - https://mydashtracker.com/

---

1. National Heart, Lung, and Blood Institute, National Institutes of Health. (2021, December 29). *The science behind the DASH eating plan.* National Heart Lung and Blood Institute. https://www.nhlbi.nih.gov/education/dash/research

2. Chauhan, V. (2023, June 8). *Using the dash diet for kidney disease: should you tweak the popular DASH diet if you have kidney disease?.* Verywell Health. https://www.verywellhealth.com/dash-diet-for-kidney-disease-does-it-work-part-1-of-2-2085845

3. Hinzey, E. (2023, September 5). *DASH diet for hypertension and healthy weight loss.* U.S. News & World Report - Health. https://health.usnews.com/best-diet/dash-diet

CHAPTER TWELVE

Mediterranean Diet

The Mediterranean Diet is an ancient, long-standing meal plan based on the diets of many countries such as Croatia, Greece, Italy, and Turkey which are located around the Mediterranean Sea. There are many versions of this diet. It is well-researched and has many health benefits for those who follow it. The benefits include longevity of life, lower cardiovascular disease, lower cancer risk, and lower risk of type 2 diabetes.[1][2]

This diet has ranked very well. It's predominately a plant-based, minimally processed diet that focuses on vegetables, fruits, whole grains nuts, and lots of healthy fats such as extra virgin olive oil. Seafood or fish is typically allowed a few times a week. Think of it this way, vegetables and fruit are your main dish and meat is a side dish. It is more than just a diet, it is a lifestyle around dining with friends and family. It can be budget-friendly as less money is spent on meat and it is known to be more conscientious for our planet. It is very flexible and can be adapted for various cultures including customizing for your halal and kosher, vegan, and vegetarian requests.

Foods to eat on this diet

- Vegetables (lots of them)

- Fruits

- Whole grains such as oats, quinoa, barley farro, rye, spelt, brown, and wild rice (my favorite is wild rice)

- Good fats such as Olives, flaxseeds, almonds, walnuts, avocadoes, and salmon

- Oils such as extra virgin olive oil sesame oil, grapeseed oil, and sunflower oil

Foods to eat in moderation:

- Some Cheeses

- Eggs

- Occasional sweets

- Pasta

- Poultry

- Red Meat

- Seafood or fish-about twice per week

- Yogurt

Foods to avoid

- Saturated and trans fats such as animal fat, butter, cocoa butter, coconut oil, dairy fat, egg yolks, fried foods, margarine, palm oil, and red meat

- Foods made with ingredients such as shortening and hydrogenated fats which are often found in cakes, cookies, donuts, pastries, and pies

- Refined carbs such as white bread and white bagels

- Highly processed meats like bacon, sausage, hot dogs, and bologna

Who is this diet best for?

- Someone who doesn't want to count carbs

- Someone who enjoys new recipes and making meals

- Someone who likes a lot of vegetables and fruit

- Someone who does not want to give up pasta

- Someone who likes to feel full (all those veggies can fill you up)

- Someone who prefers a diet that is well-researched and has health benefits

- Someone who likes flexibility in what they can eat

- Someone who wants to accommodate various cultural preferences

Who is this diet <u>not</u> best for?

- Someone who is short on time and can't do meal prep

- Someone who eats out a lot as cooking is required

- Someone who does not do well eating a lot of fat

- Someone who is not willing to incorporate more vegetables and fruits in their diet

Treats

- Occasional sweets (see "recipes" in the "resources" section)

- Occasional red wine

Robin's take on this diet

I have seen this diet make non-veggie lovers into veggie lovers. There are so many great recipes to try that are truly delicious. Also, I really like the health benefits as well. It is still important to track your calories for weight loss. I look at this diet more as a lifestyle than just a diet. It is a good way to incorporate more vegetables and fruits into your diet and possibly persuade your family members to incorporate more too! This diet does require planning, food prep, and cooking. The delicious recipes online can really make you salivate.

Resources:

- **Recipes** – *The Mediterranean Dish* website has awesome recipes. You can sort by category types such as salads, appetizers, vegetarian, desserts, etc. Also, you can look at the written recipe or video for a great "how-to". The Italian-inspired orange ricotta cake is to die for.

  - https://www.themediterraneandish.com/

- **Budget-friendly recipes:**

  - https://www.budgetbytes.com/category/recipes/global/mediterranean/

- ***The Mediterranean Dish: 120 Bold and Healthy Recipes You'll Make on Repeat: A Mediterranean* Cookbook by Suzy Karadsheh**

  - https://a.co/d/gA98Pp8

- **History of the Mediterranean Diet**

  - https://www.ncbi.nlm.nih.gov/pmc/articles/PMC3684452/

1. Martinez-Gonzalez, M. A., & Martin-Calvo, N. (2016, November). Mediterranean diet and life expectancy: beyond olive oil, fruits, and vegetables. *Current Opinion in Clinical Nutrition and Metabolic Care*, 19(6): 401-407. https://doi.org/10.1097/MCO.0000000000000316. Accessed through PubMed Central at https://www.ncbi.nlm.nih.gov/pmc/articles/PMC5902736/

2. Diabetes.co.uk. (2016, July 19). *Mediterranean diet can lower risk of type 2 diabetes, cancer and cardiovascular events*. Diabetes.co.uk - News. https://www.diabetes.co.uk/news/2016/jul/mediterranean-diet-can-lower-risk-of-type-2-diabetes,-cancer-and-cardiovascular-events-94389744.html

CHAPTER THIRTEEN

The Flexitarian Diet

The Flexitarian Diet is a semi-vegetarian diet that is primarily plant-based but has flexibility with eating occasional meat. So, if you are a gal who wants to eat healthy plant-based meals most of the time, but still wants an occasional juicy sirloin burger, then this diet may be for you. It is a low-fat diet that includes vegetables, fruits, whole grains, dairy, spices, and occasional meats. Proteins often include beans, peas, eggs, and lentils.

From a health standpoint, this diet ranks well for long-term weight loss. Plant-based diets in general tend to be helpful for heart disease, diabetes, and cancer prevention.[1]

This diet generally accommodates halal, kosher, and other dietary requests. As its name suggests, this plan is very flexible so you can phase in reducing your meat consumption over some time. It truly can be a new way of life of eating. The meal plate tends to be ½ vegetables and fruits, ¼ whole grains, and 1/4 of protein. Also, the timing of meals is not regulated so you can eat when you want.

The name *The Flexitarian Diet* was coined by dietician and author, Dawn Jackson Blatner.[2] Dawn has a great website that includes files you can save on your phone or computer and print. Files of fun stuff like ideas for a charcuterie board for a girls' night in, no-bake quick and easy dinner options, salty and sweet snack options, and even a

"Screw-Up Worksheet" if you get off track.[3] It's truly a list of fun ways to make the Flexitarian Diet part of your life. You can access Dawn's website using the following link:

https://www.dawnjacksonblatner.com/

Foods to eat on this diet

- Vegetables (lots of them)

- Fruits

- Whole grains like brown rice, quinoa

- Good fats such as olives, flaxseeds, almonds, walnuts, and avocadoes

- Oils as extra virgin olive oil, sesame oil, grapeseed oil, and sunflower oil

- Nondairy milk such as almond or oat milk

- Spices

Foods to eat in moderation

- Some Cheeses

- Eggs (an egg has 6 grams of protein per egg and 75 calories so two eggs equals 12 grams of protein and approximately 150 calories)

- Nut butters

- Occasional sweets

- Pasta

- Poultry

- Red Meat

- Seafood or fish-about twice per week (this is considered "meat" on this diet).

- Yogurt

Foods to Avoid

- Saturated and Trans-fat as animal fat, butter, cocoa butter, coconut oil, dairy fat, egg yolks, fried foods, margarine, palm oil, and red meat

- Food made with ingredients such as shortening or hydrogenated fats which are often found in cakes, cookies, donuts, pastries, and pies

- Refined carbs such as white bread and white bagels

- Highly processed meats like bacon, sausage, hot dogs, and bologna

Who is this diet best for?

- Someone who wants to incorporate more vegetables and fruits in their diet

- Someone who wants to save some money on their grocery bill. Plants in general tend to be cheaper than meat especially if you use frozen. Think of it this way, you can buy several large bags of frozen vegetables and/or fruit for what you would pay for a small pack of chicken.

- Someone who not only wants to lose weight but to also adopt a new lifestyle

- Someone who prefers a diet with researched health benefits

- Someone who likes flexibility on what they can eat as we all tend to get sick of the same old foods

- Someone who likes to eat out (although a review of the menu is important before dining)

- Someone interested in skin health, as vegetarian diets often can help with that glow[4]

- Someone who wants to follow a halal, kosher, or gluten-free diet

- Someone concerned about the environmental health of the planet

- Someone who likes to eat socially

Who is this diet <u>not</u> best for?

- Pregnant women and those with diabetes should consult with their doctor on some of the parameters for this diet

- People who don't want to incorporate more fruits and vegetables in their diet

- People who prefer a lot of structure in their diet

- People with B12 deficiency[5]

- Some people with GI issues such as bloating can have less symptoms if they eat more meat[6]

- This diet can be difficult to sustain for people who are big meat eaters

Treats

- Occasional sweets such as dark chocolate

- Occasional red wine

- Candied nuts like pecans (so yummy and smell so good!)

Robin's take on this diet

This is a great diet for women who want to transition to eating a more plant-based diet. I have found that the flexibility of this diet helps women make it a lifestyle versus just a diet and they do tend to eat healthier than they did before. Also, it is important to portion your plate to include vegetables, whole grains, and proteins. It is easy for many women to ramp up the carbs even whole grain carbs and cut back on the protein and vegetables. This diet does need to have balance. Some people will be prone to B12 deficiency since with diet is highly plant-based so it is important to consult with your doctor about supplementing with it.

This diet is really great. It often gets women to eat more vegetables and fruits, less processed food, and are healthier because of it. The flexibility makes it fun and not boring. If you are the kind of gal who likes to mix it up, not eat the same old thing, and eat lots of different foods, this is a great diet for you to try. There are a lot of great recipe resources available as well.

Resources:

Recipes:

- The Flexitarian of UK website has great recipes with videos

    - https://theflexitarian.co.uk/recipe-items/

- Dawn Blatner has great recipes and resources on her website…looking at these recipes literally makes my mouth water

    - https://www.dawnjacksonblatner.com/books/the-flexitarian-diet/flexitari an-diet-recipes/

Book:

- *The Flexitarian Diet: The Mostly Vegetarian Way to Lose Weight, Be Healthier, Prevent Disease, and Add Years to Your Life* by Dawn Jackson Blatner

    - https://a.co/d/dDCprfB

Other Resources to keep you in the know:

- Silver Dinner has Flexitarian delicious options on their menu

  - https://www.silverdiner.com/flexitarian-menu

---

1. McMacken, M., & Shah, S. (2017, May). A plant-based diet for the prevention and treatment of type 2 diabetes. *Journal of Geriatric Cardiology*, 14(5): 342-354. Accessed through PubMed Central at https://www.ncbi.nlm.nih.gov/pmc/article s/PMC5466941/

2. Frey, R. J. (n.d.). *Flexitarian diet*. Reference.Jrank.org. https://reference.jrank.org /diets/Flexitarian_Diet.html

3. Blatner, D. J. (n.d.). *Printables*. DJ Blatner. https://www.dawnjacksonblatner.co m/printables/

4. Fam, V. W., Charoenwoodhipong, P., Sivamani, R. K., Holt, R. R., Keen, C. L., & Hackman, R. M. (Epub 2021, October 30). Plant-based foods for skin health: a narrative review. *Journal of the Academy of Nutrition and Dietetics*, 2022 Mar; 122(3):614-629. Accessed through PubMed Central at https://pubmed.ncbi.nlm .nih.gov/34728412/

5. Streit, L. (2022, January 14). *The flexitarian diet*. Healthline - Nutrition. https:// www.healthline.com/nutrition/flexitarian-diet-guide

6. International Foundation for Gastrointestinal Disorders. (n.d.). *Controlling intestinal gas*. International Foundation for Gastrointestinal Disorders - GI Disorders. https://iffgd.org/gi-disorders/symptoms-causes/intestinal-gas/

CHAPTER FOURTEEN

Intermittent Fasting

The value of including intermittent fasting in our diet plan discussions is that many women have questions and have heard both good and controversial things about it and want to learn more. A big wig who has studied intermittent fasting for over 25 years is Mark Mattson Ph.D. Mark Mattson is a top neuroscientist at Johns Hopkins.[1] There have been studies with mice and rats (ick) and humans too that have had dietary restriction and it showed less degeneration in parts of the brain, weight loss, lower blood pressure, and lower cholesterol.[2]

Have I ever told you the story of when my brother was in medical school and we had rats living in cages in our basement for his research? My brother was in the early part of his medical school training and he was gathering medical statistics on a bunch of rats. The rats were in cages, but I still remember seeing those big old rat eyes looking at me when I was getting something off the shelves in the basement. So creepy!

Anyway, back to intermittent fasting, research shows that intermittent fasting can have many beneficial health benefits for your body and mind. Intermittent fasting is also known as time-restricted feeding. Intermittent fasting is more about when you eat versus what you eat. The theory is that intermittent fasting triggers the body to stop using its sugar reserves and then burn fat. It's not a bad gig if you are trying to lose weight. Dr. Mattson calls this term "metabolic switching."[3]

On this plan, snacking tends to be a no-no. By avoiding snacking, insulin levels tend to decrease and then our fat cells release stored sugar for energy.

Intermittent fasting is nothing new. Many religions follow intermittent fasting including those who observe Ramadan. There has been research comparing these religious fasting techniques with typical intermittent fasting and both are promising for longevity which can slow aging.[4]

How it works?

There are many ways you can do intermittent fasting. Here are the typical plans.

Eat in an 8-hour window

You can eat all of your meals within an 8-hour window and then fast for 16 hours. This may sound difficult, but it is not as difficult as you think. An example is if you get up at 7 a.m. and have a cup of coffee, tea or water and then eat at 10 a.m. Then you can eat anytime up until 6 pm. This plan is often one big meal or two meals a day. After 6 pm, the kitchen (and TV room) is closed, and you can't eat until the next day at 10 am. Other options that people like are eating between 11 a.m. and 7 p.m. so they can eat lunch and dinner or eating between 12 p.m. and 8 p.m. One thing to note is that it is a good habit to not eat too close to bedtime. I have found that, at first, many people find this difficult, but then they find a routine that works best for them.

Eat in a 12-hour window

This is the same as above, but you eat your meals within a 12-hour window. One option is you could eat between 7 a.m. and 7 p.m.

Alternate fasting

With this type of intermittent fasting, you eat your typical 3 meals a day for 5 days and then 2 days per week would restrict calories to around 600. Many people find that it is easier to do their "fasting days" during the week when they are busy versus on the weekends when they eat out more and have less of a routine. For example, you can do calorie-restricted fasting on Mondays and Tuesdays and then eat 3 meals a day for the rest of the week.

Important: Just remember to lose weight you still need to watch your calories and the types of foods you eat.

What can you eat with intermittent fasting?

- Vegetables including potatoes

- Fruits including avocados

- Whole grains

- Lean Protein as poultry, turkey, fish, and seafood

- Lentils and Beans

- Nuts and Seeds

- Eggs

What foods to avoid?

- High-sugar foods such as cakes, cookies, and pies

- High-salt foods such as frozen dinner meals, chips, and pretzels

What can you drink on intermittent fasting?

- Water

- Water with lemon

- Mineral Water

- No-sugar beverages like flavored seltzers

- Coffee-black

- Tea-black

What drinks not to drink during intermittent fasting?

- Alcohol (sorry gals)

- Coconut water

- Milk

- Sodas

- Diet Sodas -artificial sweeteners can sometimes affect your insulin levels

Who is this diet good for?

- Someone who is concerned about brain health, especially cognitive and memory decline

- Someone who focuses on longevity

- Someone who is concerned about heart health, especially their blood pressure

- Type 2 diabetics (with doctor supervision)

- Someone who likes to focus on athletic performance

- Someone with certain types of digestive issues. The theory here is that it gives your digestive system a break from eating often. I have found this very helpful for me with my digestive issues.

Who is this diet <u>not</u> good for?

- Children under 18-year-old as they are still growing

- Pregnant and breastfeeding women

- Type 1 Diabetics

- Those with Eating Disorders

- Someone who often gets "hangry"

- Someone who tends to get "shaky" or weak when they don't eat at regular planned times

- Someone who won't give up snacking or grazing

Robin's take on this

Many people do well with intermittent fasting, but it should be very individualized. Often, it takes some time to get used to make it a habit. I have known some women who have symptoms such as weakness, shakiness, fatigue, low blood pressure, and fainting where intermittent fasting is not the best for them. I recommend reviewing your medical history with your doctor and then asking them if they think intermittent fasting is a good option for you.

It is important to consider is how many calories you are consuming. To lose weight you do need to reduce your calories so if you eat 4,500 plus calorie meals in an 8-hour window frame you will almost be guaranteed to not lose weight. For me personally, I have found that intermittent fasting is very helpful with my digestive issues. I was a breakfast smoothie kind of gal, but now I typically wait until lunchtime to eat my first meal. Also, remember that it is still important that you eat quality food such as vegetables, fruits, whole grains, and lean protein.

Booze is another issue. If you have fasted and then drink alcohol on an empty stomach it will metabolize differently than if you had eaten. Beware as Tipsy Turvey, can happen quicker than you think. So keep in mind, it is best to avoid alcohol when you are fasting.

Resources:

- **Learn more about Mark Mattson, Ph.D.**

    - https://neuroscience.jhu.edu/research/faculty/57

- **Documentary - Eat Fast, Live Longer**

    - https://www.youtube.com/watch?v=Ihhj_VSKiTs

- **Book -*The Obesity Code* by Dr. Jason Fong**

    - https://a.co/d/80aysUb

---

1. Wikipedia. (2023, October 9). *Mark Mattson.* https://en.wikipedia.org/wiki/Mark_Mattson

2. Mattson, M. P., Longo, V. D., & Harvie, M. (2016, October 31). *Impact of intermittent fasting on health and disease processes.* PubMed Central. https://www.ncbi.nlm.nih.gov/pmc/articles/PMC5411330/

3. Mattson, M., & Patrick, R. (2021, October 6). *Dr. Mark Mattson on the benefits of stress, metabolic switching, fasting, and hormesis.* FoundMyFitness. https://www.foundmyfitness.com/episodes/mark-mattson

4. Hoddy, K. K., Marlatt, K. L., Çetinkaya, H., & Ravussin, E. (2020, July). *Intermittent fasting and metabolic health: From religious fast to time-restricted feeding.* PubMed Central. https://www.ncbi.nlm.nih.gov/pmc/articles/PMC7419159/

CHAPTER FIFTEEN

Migraine Diet

If you are a migraine sufferer like me (yuck, I have had them since age 11!) you may want to check out this dietary plan. Angela Stanton, PhD is the founder of this plan and is a researcher, neuroeconomist, and author.[1]

Dr. Stanton, herself, is also a migraine sufferer and the author of the book, *Fighting the Migraine Epidemic.* She has a large Facebook group where she will answer your questions. This diet is a very high-fat, low-carb diet that includes dairy. It is quite detailed hence terming the name protocol. You need to like to eat meat as it is a more carnivore-style diet. If you are interested, I recommend checking out the book and looking at the PDF and guide files on the Facebook group. The Facebook group pdf files educate on multiple topics including recipes and tips on what to do when flying if the barometric pressure is changing to avoid a migraine.

Resources:

- **Book: *Fighting the Migraine Epidemic: A Complete Guide – How to Treat and Prevent Migraines Without Medicine,* by Angela A. Stanton, Ph.D.**

- https://a.co/d/57NPDyA

- **Migraine Facebook Group – "Migraine Sufferers Who Want to Heal by the Stanton Migraine Protocol"**

  - https://www.facebook.com/groups/219182458276615

  - **Facebook Group Guides** — https://www.facebook.com/groups/Migrai neSufferers/file

---

1. Stanton, A. A. (n.d.). *Angela A. Stanton PhD*. LinkedIn. https://www.linkedin.com/in/angelaastantonphd

CHAPTER SIXTEEN

Putting it All Together

By now you have reviewed the various diets and you have found one that you prefer. Moving forward here is some helpful information.

Diet Tips

Eat foods you like

I have seen this over and over again; a girlfriend has a friend who lost a lot of weight on a particular diet and wants to try it so she can lose weight too. After a short time, she decided that the diet didn't work for her, and no weight loss was achieved. One of the keys to starting a weight loss plan is to eat food that you like. If you hate broccoli or Brussels sprouts, then don't worry about eating them. If you love carrots and celery sticks, go for it. Dieting is tough enough without trying a bunch of new foods. Start by eating foods that you already like. I've included a list of grocery items in the "Resources" section of this chapter that you might find helpful. Circle the foods you like and put them in your grocery cart.

Acknowledge your stress

This is a big one that has taken me years to figure out. For a long time, I would eat a lot of salads and eat fairly healthy (except for a few treats from Rita's and Dunkin) and still not lose weight. At one point in my life, I was dealing with chronic stress. The kind of stress that just won't go away as much as I wish it did. Stress when the big things happen like grief, divorce, medical issues, challenges with our children or grandchildren, severe money concerns, etc. It was especially difficult for me after adopting my son. In some time, I came to have self-realization that I needed to get my stress under control. In my case, I needed to get breaks from my situation so that I could recharge and restore my energy. After I got my stress under control, I had much better success with my weight loss. Reducing my cortisol levels was a key component of my success.

Staying on Track

How do you keep yourself motivated to continue on your new plan? I have found that many women start a new diet, but have a hard time sticking to it for more than a week or two. Here are some tips I have found along the way to keep your motivation and gusto up.

Reward yourself for small successes along the way

I'm not talking about a hot fudge sundae here but rewarding yourself with a non-food item or experience. Perhaps you haven't had your nails done in a long time or you want to buy yourself a new blouse at Kohl's, Target, or Walmart. Maybe life has been stressful and you schedule a massage. It doesn't have to be expensive items, you could reserve an eBook or book from the library and sit with a cup of warm coffee and peacefully read. You can walk a favorite trail and take pictures of flowers and wildlife with your phone. Whatever it is, pat yourself on the back and acknowledge your effort, your effort of being persistent and consistent!

Positive affirmations

It is so easy to get caught up in negativity by thinking and feeling negative thoughts. I remember when I was getting my master's degree, there was a term called *negativity bias* and the instructor discussed how positive thoughts slide off like Teflon and negative thoughts stick and don't let go. Each day, try writing in a journal and then speak your thoughts out loud (this helps you retain things better). Say things like "I can do this", "my health will be better when I do this", or "I am hopeful". Be sure to make it personal to you.

Plan

Plan for success. Set aside one day a week when you can plan for the upcoming week. For example, on Sundays, you can shop for groceries or have them delivered, cut up vegetables and fruits for the week (or use frozen), and write out on your phone or notebook meal plan ideas. This way you are making it easier for yourself throughout the week. No excuses that you don't have food in the house, and you need to call for a pizza or you just don't know what to make for dinner. Spending an hour or two on one day and having a plan will make your entire week better.

Have short-term goals

I remember years ago when I needed to lose over 100 pounds. I kept making big goals like trying to lose 20 pounds at a time. My intentions were noble, but my goals were too big. Shoot for smaller goals like losing 2 pounds in a week or 5 pounds in 2 weeks. These are more realistic goals that you can visualize and you are more likely to realistically achieve them.

Ask loved ones to support you

There are going to be loved ones who are food pushers. They bug you to eat one more slice of pizza, even though you say you are full or "are hurt" that you didn't have a slice of their delicious homemade pie. Don't go to these people for support in your weight loss healthy eating plan. Instead, go to your girlfriends and loved ones who you trust and ask them to hold you accountable. Ask them to call you out if you are not complying or ask how you are feeling. Support from these loved ones makes a big difference. Even better, you may have a girlfriend or loved one who wants to do the plan with you. Having a buddy on your weight loss journey is very helpful.

Movement

You don't have to be a marathon runner or speed skater. Just make it a point to move your body each day. During your Netflix or TV watching time, set your cell phone alarm to get up at commercial breaks or pauses and do some jumping jacks, sit-ups, leg lifts, or arm circles If you have a condition like a bad knee, you can still do arm circles. If you can't jump, you can still do leg lifts. Don't blame one medical issue for not letting you move other parts of your body. Ask your doctor for which exercises are good for you to do. YouTube has many videos to watch once you decide the kind of movement you want to do. Remember, not only is movement good for burning calories but it is great for your brain too! And remember, the more muscle in your body, the more calories you burn.

How to avoid food temptations?

It is not uncommon for all of us to have cravings for that tall Latte, a big bowl of ice cream, or popcorn. You may have seen an ad on TV where that pumpkin spice latte or that chocolate caramel drink looks oh-so-good and you're finding it hard to resist. Here are some tips I have learned along the way to help.

Make a healthier version of what you are craving

So say you are craving that pumpkin spice latte, look online at recipes by Joy Bauer or Dr. Axe and search "pumpkin" to see what recipes pop up. There are so many recipes to choose from and they are delicious too! Usually, you can find the calorie and nutritional information too. Many of the recipes don't have a lot of ingredients, are easy to prepare, and save you some bucks too!

Remind yourself of the negatives

This is one time where I am telling you not to be so positive. Say things to yourself like "After that tall latte I feel wired and then tired" or "I feel bloated after that tall latte" or "That latte has more calories than I am allocated for half my day, it's not worth it". Acknowledge your feelings and then pat yourself on the back for having the willpower to pass by that Donut or coffee drive-thru this time.

Distractions

When you are having a craving, pause and think about doing something else for a while. Perhaps you can play a game on your phone, catch up with a girlfriend on the phone or via text, start a craft project or listen to some great music. Oftentimes, when I need a distraction, I will ask Alexa to play my favorite song list and sing along or dance.

What to do if you get off track?

It's your birthday and you were only going to eat one bite of cake. Your girlfriend or sister put so much time and effort into making the cake that you didn't want to be rude, so you ate lots of it and before you know it you ate half the cake. And to top it off, afterward, you had a few extra glasses of wine. The next day you feel guilty, and you splurge too because you feel bad. On Monday, you go to work and you see the donuts and you think "What the heck, I blew it this weekend, why not eat them too?"

Remind yourself that we all get off track sometimes. Stuff happens, emotions can run high, and stressful situations occur. The best thing to do is to acknowledge what happened, forgive yourself, and then recommit to your goals. Brainstorm with yourself or a friend on how to do things differently next time in a similar situation. For example, have a small slice of cake and then move it to another room so you don't see it.

Stress Release

A lot of times we get off track because we are stressed. We sometimes self-medicate with that extra glass of wine or pint of ice cream. The key is to find more healthy productive ways to manage our stress. Things like walking, singing out loud, or spending time with friends are some examples.

We all have that friend who gets off track in life whether it is with their diet or a personal matter that likes to consistently tell everyone over and over again how they screwed up. Don't be that person! It's okay to acknowledge you had a setback and tell a friend or loved one but don't keep repeating it over and over again. Give your brain a rest and spend your brain power moving forward not backward. Think of it this way, like the great Michael Jackson song, "I'm starting with the man (woman in this case) in the mirror [...] take a look at yourself and then make a change."

Seek help if you need it

I have known some girlfriends who despite their best efforts, consistently just can't get back on track. Sometimes they may have an undiagnosed condition such as ADHD, OCD, or anxiety. Getting therapy is easier than ever now, especially with remote services. Also, funding is more available than ever for those who don't have therapy funds in their budget. There are many good types of therapy like Cognitive Behavioral Therapy and DBT. There are, also, great supplements and medications that can help too! Feel free to email me if you want some resources for this.

Reasons why diets fail?

Sleep

You can eat all the carrots in the world, but if you can't sleep, you can lose your focus on tasks during the day which can make complying with the diet very difficult. You may feel groggy, fatigued, and a tad cranky. Sleep is a big issue for many people especially women as they age. Either women can't fall asleep, they can't stay asleep, their mind has a difficult time shutting down (oh that racing brain with so much stuff to do) or they wake up way too early like at 4 am instead of 6 am. I can't tell you how many women I have talked to who have had a pattern of sleep issues that have lasted for years. I am not talking about the occasional sleepless night, I'm talking about that most nights they have sleep issues. If you are one of those people, please check out this section of the book. First, we'll dive into good sleep etiquette and then things to try that you may have not tried in the past before.

Sleep Etiquette Tips

Winding Down

I often hear women say that they just can't turn their brains off at night. They are worried about their kids, grandkids, nieces, nephews, jobs, finances, to-do lists, etc. If this is you, you are not alone. To wind down to get your body and mind ready for restorative sleep and some good Z's by taking a warm bath with Epsom salt, reading, journaling, or listening to calming music. Take some time to do stress-free activities. If you do read from your cell phone or tablet, turn the brightness down on the settings. Do not engage in paying bills, looking at finances, problem-solving, competitive games, or sports just before bedtime.

Several years ago, I unexpectedly and tragically lost one of my sons. It was the most emotionally devasting time in my life. I was emotionally and physically exhausted and needed to sleep yet still had difficulty falling asleep. I never really had sleep issues until this time. My dear cousin gave me a journal to write in and I started to write in it every morning and evening. Much to my surprise, it helped me relax and fall asleep even though it was a very tough time. Journalling worked for me. Reading helped too. Doing quiet activities can help establish or get back to sleep routines again.

Make a good sleep environment

A cool (not freezing), dark room is often the best for sleep. If your blinds are not "blackout blinds" you may want to get some. The darker the better. Also, keep noise to a minimum.

If your partner snores or there is traffic noise, consider getting earplugs. Turn your ringer down on your cell phone. Remind your family and friends not to interrupt you while you are sleeping to keep interruptions down. Keep interruptions for emergencies only.

Use your bedroom for sleep and romance only[1]

You may have piles to go through in your bedroom or things to put away. Consider putting those piles in a closet or another room temporarily and perhaps leaving the TV out of your room. Get them out of your sight. Focus on keeping the rest of your life out of the bedroom and use it for sleep and romance only. Everything else can wait. This is a big one that psychologists often mention to patients.

Keep a consistent sleep routine

If during the week you sleep from 10:30 p.m. to 6:30 a.m., try to do that most of the time. It is tempting to sleep in on the weekends, but it really is important that your body knows that it is bedtime and that you allocate at least 7 hours or so to sleep excluding falling asleep time. This may take some discipline, but your body will start remembering your bedtime and help you get some shut-eye.

Avoid caffeine near bedtime

You may have been out to a café and had a decaf coffee and found you couldn't fall asleep that night. Spoiler alert, some decaf coffees have caffeine in them. If you are sensitive to caffeine, avoid caffeine near bedtime. Some people need to avoid it within 5 hours of bedtime and others can only do caffeine in the morning. Reflect on your caffeine patterns to determine if you can have any or when to have it.

Avoid booze near bedtime

Although alcohol may help you fall asleep initially it can actually disrupt sleep. Therefore, be sure to keep that glass of wine to earlier in the evening.

Do Physical Activity, but not too close to bedtime

I always sleep better on days when I have walked with a friend or biked a few miles. You don't need to run a marathon or swim in an Olympic-sized pool, but it is important to get some activity in your day. It might be something like playing catch with your dog, doing yoga while watching a YouTube video, or walking a few times to the mailbox. By the way, yoga is really beneficial because it is good for your mind, body, and spirit and tends to be meditative which is important near bedtime. Whatever it is, physical movement can help with sleep. Just be sure not to do it too close to bedtime.

When all else fails

- **Warm your tummy** – Your mom may have given you a warm hot water bottle to use when you were a child. This is the same concept, put the warm compress on your belly area and relax, and enjoy the warmth. Be sure to take it off before you slumber.

- **Take a Sleep Master Class** – Dr. Hyman has a free one. You can access it at: https://courses.drhyman.com/sleep-course-own

- **If melatonin has not worked for you** – Try to supplement with passion-flower[2] or with Valerian[3]

- **Leg or body cramps**? Try using magnesium spray or take a magnesium supplement[4]

- **Ask your doctor to check your Vitamin D levels and see if you need to supplement with it** There is extensive research now showing that low Vitamin D levels are associated with poor sleep.[5] Vitamin D is easy to supplement with. Also, research has shown that low levels of Vitamin D are associated with obesity.[6] Lastly, remember that Vitamin D is a fat-soluble vitamin so eating fat with it can aid with absorption.[7]

If all else fails, contact your insurance company or local health department and **ask for a sleep evaluation and a referral to a specialist**. **Don't let this go on,** you can improve your sleep! Be sure to document your issue before going to your appointment. Can you not fall asleep? Not stay asleep? Can't sleep at all? Your mind races? Or, do you wake up too early? Does your sleep differ from what you ate that day? **Be specific**. Observe yourself and take this information to the sleep specialist.

Important!
Be sure to consult with your doctor before using any new supplements.

Stress Management

You may have been working too many hours, missing your family and friends, are lonely, bored, or are going through a difficult relationship or financial time. Or perhaps you are dealing with the grief of losing a parent, a spouse, or a loved one. Let's face it! Life can really get stressful and it doesn't always go the way we had hoped, planned, and dreamed of. There were multiple times in my life when life got extremely hard, and the stress was extremely elevated and felt unbearable. One time was after we adopted my son and he came home with numerous unforeseen issues. The other is when I lost my oldest son when he was 20 years old. I can't say I am an expert on stress management, but I can say I have experienced significant stress and can relate to some of the things you are going through.

Here are some tips for managing stress.

The perception of stress can feel as bad as the stress itself[8]

You may be worried about what will happen to your son if he never gets a job or won't stop playing video games, or you may be praying your daughter can get pregnant or you may be concerned about what happens if a medical condition returns again. Have you noticed how fear of "what ifs" can really hurt and dive deep into your soul? Whatever the stress, the worry can really take its toll on our minds, bodies, and souls. So, with that being said, how do we cope during the difficult times? Take a moment to acknowledge and be with your feelings and emotions. Have some self-compassion and then continue to focus on your life and acknowledge that you cannot control everything that happens. Focus on the things you can control and try not to continue repeating how you feel to yourself in your mind. It's okay to tell a close friend or confidant how you're feeling but don't repeat it 10 times a day to 10 different people. It just isn't healthy to stay in that emotional state for an extended time. This is easier said than done but if you become self-aware that all your brainpower is being focused on the stress you can redirect emotions to be more at peace.

Physical Movement

You may have heard that physical activity is good for your heart, but it is also good for your mind. After I lost my son there were days when it was difficult to even get out of bed. I was miserable and really didn't even want to face the world. A friend suggested that I should walk daily even if it was only to the mailbox. I started doing this and eventually, I started walking a lot. It got me out of the house and out of my head. On my walks, I would see birds and flowers and the world being active. It really did help me get through some difficult times. If walking isn't your thing, there are many other things to try. Perhaps doing a yoga or Pilates class at the YMCA, watching and exercising to a video online, or playing a sport like pickleball. It can even be unstructured activities like taking the stairs, doing 25 sit-ups or 10 girl pushups each day. Even chair yoga is fun to do while watching TV during the commercials. The key is to decide what movement to do daily and then set short goals for yourself. Don't just think about it, do it.

Do more of the things that bring you peace and you love and enjoy to do

This is a great time in our lives to do more of the things that we really enjoy doing that bring us contentment and peace. It may be taking up crafts that you used to do as painting, crocheting, or making beautiful holiday ornaments. It may be exploring beautiful destinations online or places that you would like to travel. It may be sitting in solitude on a brisk morning or evening and reading your favorite book. It may be taking a sewing, baking, or other fun class in person or online. Take a moment now and think and write about the things you would love to do. List three on the lines that follow ...

1. _______________________________________

2. _______________________________________

3. _______________________________________

This is something I used after I lost my eldest son, I really felt I needed to find some things to do that calmed my emotions. I found that reading books that I found interesting helped as well as journalling and doing crafts. I didn't always finish everything, but it did get me out of my own mind and calmed me during that very awful time. Volunteering and seeing through the eyes of others can help too!

The key is not only to plan things you like to do but to schedule time to do them. It may be a Saturday afternoon or a weekday evening instead of watching TV or surfing the net. Grab your online calendar on your phone or your calendar on your wall and schedule the activities that restore your soul.

These kinds of activities refer to the term "flow"[9] and is often used in positive psychology (which is something I am a big believer in), and it has helped me personally get through some tough times. If you are interested in learning more about it, I have listed some resources below on positive psychology.

Seek guidance if need be

This is a big one. Life can get complicated. You may have had some trauma in your life, are dealing with grief, had sexual abuse, experienced discrimination, have anxiety or attention issues, or perhaps some addiction issues. It is not uncommon for us to self-medicate with food, alcohol, marijuana, other drugs, excessive shopping, excessive sex (not just men gals), etc. Whatever your guilty pleasure is, don't be too hard on yourself. Life can get hard and complicated. You may need assistance from a mental health provider who can help you break the cycle to live a more peaceful and meaningful life.

I have done quite a bit of health education in the mental health field including getting to know psychiatrists, psychologists, licensed clinical social workers, etc. I have worked on programs on things such as screen, drug and alcohol, and opioid addictions. If you feel you are ready to seek help, there really is more flexibility in scheduling online and in-person counseling appointments than ever before. There, are also, well-researched medications and supplements available that can help as well. The medication thing is not a popular choice for a health coach to promote, as we often try to manage health more naturally. However, I have really seen it help get women back on track. Also, there is more funding available than ever for mental health due to some of the big settlements with pharmaceutical companies.[10] If cost is an issue for you, feel free to contact me and I can help you find some local resources.

Friend, for you to live your best life both emotionally and physically, take that first step and commit to seeking help. **Don't just think about it, DO IT!** Your mind, body, and spirit will be better for it.

Other Stress Busters

There are many other options that can be used to combat stress. These stress busters include expressing gratitude, volunteering, fostering relationships, acceptance, positive self-talk, and more. One day I will probably write a book focused just on that topic for women our age.

Resources:

- **Grocery List** - You can find the grocery list I mentioned at the start of this chapter at the following link: https://www.wellnessgirlfriend.com/which-diet-is-best-for-me

- **Positive Psychology** – Here are some great TED talks on positive psychology. Martin Seligman in particular is known to be an expert in this field: https://positivepsychology.com/positive-psychology-ted-talks/

- **Authentic Happiness** – You can also go to Martin Seligman's website to learn more: https://www.authentichappiness.sas.upenn.edu/

- **Self-Compassion** – Kristin Neff is an expert on self-compassion. Isn't it true that sometimes we are our own worst critic? She has some great online events. Anyway, if you are interested in learning more about this topic, here is her website: https://self-compassion.org/

---

1. The National Institute for Occupational Safety and Health. (2020, March 31). *NIOSH training for nurses on shift work and long work hours, part 2. strategies to reduce risks, module 6. improving your sleep and alertness: create a good sleep environment (continued)*. Centers for Disease Control and Prevention. https://www.cdc.gov/niosh/work-hour-training-for-nurses/longhours/mod6/03.html

2. Suni, E., & Rehman, A. (2023, October 5). *Natural sleep aids*. Sleep Foundation. https://www.sleepfoundation.org/sleep-aids/natural-sleep-aids

3. Summer, J., & Singh, A. (2023, November 8). *Valerian root: Sleep benefits and side effects*. Sleep Foundation. https://www.sleepfoundation.org/sleep-aids/valerian-root

4. Jennings, K.-A. (2017, April 30). *Does magnesium help you sleep better?*. Healthline. https://www.healthline.com/nutrition/magnesium-and-sleep#what-is-magnesium

5. Abboud, M. (2022, March 3). *Vitamin D supplementation and sleep: A systematic review and meta-analysis of intervention studies*. PubMed Central. https://www.ncbi.nlm.nih.gov/pmc/articles/PMC8912284/

6. Apovian, C. (2022, December 27). *Does vitamin D deficiency cause obesity or vice versa?*. Medscape. https://www.medscape.com/viewarticle/985973?form=fpf

7. Examine.com. (n.d.). *How much fat do I need to absorb vitamin D?*. Examine. https://examine.com/supplements/vitamin-d/faq/how-much-fat-do-i-need-to-absorb-vitamin-d/

8. Keller, A., Litzelman, K., Wisk, L. E., Maddox, T., Cheng, E. R., Creswell, P. D., & Witt, W. P. (2011, December 26). *Does the perception that stress affects health matter? The association with health and mortality.* PubMed Central. https://www.ncbi.nlm.nih.gov/pmc/articles/PMC3374921/

9. Nash, J. (2019, April 11). *6 Flow Activities & Training: How to achieve a flow state.* PositivePsychology.com. https://positivepsychology.com/flow-activities/

10. Johns Hopkins Bloomberg School of Public Health. (n.d.). *Principles for the use of funds from the opioid litigation: Nationally recognized guidance for opioid settlement funds.* Opioid Principles. https://opioidprinciples.jhsph.edu/

CHAPTER SEVENTEEN

It's a Wrap!

In closing, I am so happy you took the time and initiative to read this book and to work on improving your health and well-being. Give yourself a pat on the back or a high five for wanting to improve your wellness. This book has been a pleasure to write for you. As women, it is really wonderful that we can collaborate with each other on what works for us as we age. Embracing aging to live our best life is truly a blessing.

Feel free to reach out to me at Robin@WellnessGirfriend.com or on the Facebook group https://www.facebook.com/groups/1256302791704215 I would really like to hear from you on what diet you decided to do, your progress, and how you are embracing aging.

Be Well and Take Care,

Robin